THROUGH THE LOOKING GLASS

GLASS

DIAGNOSING AND TREATING LONG COVID
USING THE PERRIN TECHNIQUE

In memory of

A caring and loving Perrin Technique™ practitioner

Ruth Wolstenholme

1977–2023

&

My dear friend, and philanthropist for ME/CFS causes

Dr Andrew Douglas PhD

1960–2023

&

A true medical pioneer in the field of ME/CFS and Lyme disease

Friend, mentor and colleague

Dr Andy Wright

1959–2024

THROUGH THE LOOKING GLASS

GLASS

DIAGNOSING AND TREATING LONG COVID
USING THE PERRIN TECHNIQUE

DR RAYMOND PERRIN

DO PhD

Osteopath and Neuroscientist

Foreword by Dr Yassine Bendiabdallah

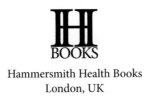

Hammersmith Health Books
London, UK

First published in 2024 by Hammersmith Health Books
– an imprint of Hammersmith Books Limited
4/4A Bloomsbury Square, London WC1A 2RP, UK
www.hammersmithbooks.co.uk

The information contained in this book is for educational purposes only. It is the result of the study and the experience of the author. Whilst the information and advice offered are believed to be true and accurate at the time of going to press, neither the author nor the publisher can accept any legal responsibility or liability for any errors or omissions that may have been made or for any adverse effects which may occur as a result of following the recommendations given herein. Always consult a qualified medical practitioner if you have any concerns regarding your health.

British Library Cataloguing in Publication Data: A CIP record of this book is available from the British Library.

Print ISBN 978-1-78161-256-9
Ebook ISBN 978-1-78161-257-6

Commissioning editor: Georgina Bentliff
Designed and typeset by: Julie Bennett of Bespoke Publishing Ltd
Cover design by: Madeline Meckiffe
Index: Dr Laurence Errington
Production: Angela Young
Printed and bound by: TJ Books Ltd, Cornwall, UK
Images: ShiipArt/Shutterstock

Contents

List of illustrations

Chapter 5: The recovery process

Chapter 6: Can long COVID be cured?

Chapter 7: Self-help advice

Chapter 9: Diet and supplements

Appendix: Frequently asked questions

Colour plates (opposite page 166)

Chapter quotations

The quotations that open each chapter are all taken from:

    Carroll, L. (2016) *Alice In Wonderland Collection: All Four Books*. Los Angeles, CA: Enhanced Media.

Acknowledgements

'Appreciation is a wonderful thing. It makes what is excellent in others belong to us as well.'

Voltaire

Thanks to my colleagues and all the amazing patients, plus their families and friends, who over the years have increased awareness of my work and raised most of the funds for my continued research. There have been so many kind donations and hundreds of wonderful people who have organised dinners, dances and musical evenings, jogged hundreds of miles, climbed mountains, cycled in cartoon outfits, walked in deep-sea diver suits, swum lakes and kayaked down mountain rivers, all to help pay the costs for the previous and ongoing scientific studies that are needed to further understand how the Perrin Technique™ can help the millions of sufferers of ME/CFS, fibromyalgia and now long COVID.

Thanks to my clinical team in Manchester, Bushey and Chalfont, Ian Totter, Sylveen Monaghan, Antoinette Atuah, Sophie King and Rakhee Mediratta. The clinic and all the work that goes on behind the scenes is run by the most important person in the practice, Elaine Coleman, who has been the most amazing practice manager for the bulk of the years I have been treating ME/CFS.

To Liv McDonald with support from Jess Stafford who are the most helpful and necessary support for the increasing worldwide network of licensed Perrin Technique™ practitioners. Thanks to Liv for the illuminating monthly practitioner newsletter sent out to all corners of the globe and her ever-expanding role as VP Perrin Technique™ Global which includes international patient liaison officer for the Perrin Technique™. Liv also brilliantly narrated the self-help guide which featured patients Georgia Morrey and Clark Geden, thanks to them all for a perfect job and to director Jonathan Rose plus his film crew for their skilful production.

A special thanks to the past and present trustees of the Fund for Osteopathic Research into ME (FORME Trust) for all their continuous help and support with my long COVID projects especially the Chair, Bev McDonald, and past and present treasurers Tina Rushton and Mags Connoly-Park, and practitioners

Laurent Heib and Ian Trotter.

An extra special mention for the amazing Dr Ruby Tam, DO in Minneapolis who has established the world's first charity-funded free clinic offering the Perrin Technique™, and profound appreciation for the continuing incredible fund-raising efforts of Perrin Technique™ practitioner Sue Capstick and her team of physiotherapists, friends and family who annually take part and offer treatments for the runners in the Wigan 10 k event.

Thanks again to my most wonderful publisher Georgina Bentliff, and her excellent team at Hammersmith Health Books, especially the most diligent editor Carolyn White, who has again helped turn my scientific ramblings into a readable book.

My utmost gratitude to a rising star in functional medicine, Yassine, for helping promote my work in the scientific and medical world and for his beautiful foreword for this book.

Thanks to my new American friends Catherine, Leslyn, Matt, Siobhan, Gail, Jen and Kelly of Lipedema Simplified and The Lipedema Project for their knowledge and resources in helping me unlock the mysteries of these and other central lymphatic disorders.

Thanks also to my magnificent research team at The University of Manchester, Adrian Heald, Mark Hann and Lisa Riste who went above and beyond the call of duty to complete our long COVID study with the NHS on time and within budget. Also, a very special thanks to Lisa for her help in keeping the self-help advice intelligible and for her beautiful poem at the beginning of this book, plus a special mention and thanks to Chris for all you have done and plan to do in the future in helping me reach my goals.

Thanks also to Dr Lewis Bass DO for his gift of neodymium magnet discs and patient advocate Catherine Vandome who suggested that the magnets might identify metals in her body, which helped the new discovery of magnetic thoracic spines in many of my patients.

And last but not least, my family. Julie, I couldn't have achieved anything without your love and support. To Jonny, Max and Josh I'm so proud of all that you have and will hopefully achieve in the future, and finally remembering my dearest mum and dad, resting together forever in peace.

Ray Perrin

Foreword

My introduction to the Perrin Technique™ came through a patient undergoing treatment for long COVID. As a practitioner of functional medicine, my initial encounter with this condition wasn't by choice but rather due to my own experience with it in late March 2020. Amidst the uncertainty surrounding long COVID during that time, I found myself revisiting my knowledge on effective approaches for post-viral infections, which I commonly address in my practice. However, I sensed a gap in my usual strategies utilised for conditions like ME/CFS or post-viral co-infections. Though I managed to regain some functionality, I still felt something was amiss. It wasn't until my patient suggested the Perrin Technique™ that I decided to explore it further. Intrigued, I underwent my first session and soon realised its efficacy. While I had previously recommended lymphatic drainage or cranial osteopathy for toxin relief to my patients, the Perrin Technique™ offered a more comprehensive, evidence-based approach that proved highly effective in combating this debilitating condition. It has since become an indispensable tool in my arsenal of therapies for long COVID.

Dr Perrin draws upon over 30 years of research and clinical expertise in managing and treating conditions like ME/CFS and post-viral syndromes, sharing his insights in his latest book. His foresight into the post-viral syndrome following SARS-CoV-2 infection was evident in a letter he sent to the *Medical Hypotheses* journal in March, 2020, entitled: 'Into the Looking Glass: Post-viral Syndrome Post COVID-19'. This letter, eventually published in June 2020, forms the backbone of his book.

Dr Perrin's book includes a clear and engaging exploration of the Perrin Technique™, laying the foundation for readers with essential concepts that will guide them through other chapters. Each chapter is enriched by a compelling, real-life patient account, offering invaluable insights into their journey to recovery with the Perrin Technique™. In the initial chapters, Dr Perrin elucidates the complexities of long COVID, the significance of detoxification, and the progressive stages leading to this condition. This pivotal account often sparks moments of revelation for readers, providing answers to the perplexing question: 'Why me?'

Chapter 4 marks a turning point, as readers gain a deeper understanding of the interplay between the glymphatic system, toxin accumulation and the role of the hypothalamus. Dr Perrin then introduces the 10-step Perrin Technique™ (page 105), tailored for Perrin-trained practitioners, alongside self-massage techniques for patients to utilise between treatments (Chapter 7: Self-help advice). This chapter serves as a practical roadmap toward recovery, offering both professionals and patients alike invaluable tools for managing long COVID effectively.

In Chapter 5, informed by what Dr Perrin calls the 'jigsaw puzzle analogy', he paints a vivid picture of the road to recovery using this useful metaphor. He illustrates how various techniques contribute to rebuilding this jigsaw puzzle piece by piece, with the Perrin Technique™ forming the essential edges. Additionally, he outlines methods for scoring patients based on their symptoms and presentation, providing a comprehensive framework for treatment.

Chapter 8 explores additional strategies for managing long COVID, including a discussion of alternative approaches that may prove successful.

In the final chapter, Dr Perrin offers a compelling summary, providing readers with a glimpse into the real-life experience of a patient with long COVID over a 24-hour period. He also shares occupational strategies that can prove beneficial, as well as cautioning which measures to avoid, offering valuable insights for navigating life with long COVID.

Overall, this book serves as a beacon of hope for patients and practitioners alike seeking to understand long COVID and the Perrin Technique™. It is rich with information supported by the latest research, appealing to both academic and curious readers alike. With its detailed approach, it provides a roadmap for overcoming this often misunderstood and debilitating condition.

Dr Yassine Bendiabdallah MPharm, PhD, IP, ABAAHP, FAAMM
Co-Founder of ZEN Healthcare, London

Dr Yassine Bendiabdallah is a Functional Medicine Specialist celebrated for his expertise in Longevity, Bio-identical Hormone Replacement Therapy (BHRT), and Post Viral Fatigue Syndrome (PVFS).

With a background as an anticancer research scientist at Cancer Research UK at University College London, Dr Bendiabdallah has gained numerous accolades and has made significant contributions to peer-reviewed academic journals. His clinical focus encompasses personalised nutrition, myalgic encephalomyelitis/ chronic fatigue syndrome (ME/CFS), longevity strategies and hormonal optimization therapies.

As the co-founder of ZEN Healthcare, a leading health and wellness centre with multiple locations across London, Dr Bendiabdallah currently serves as the Medical Director. In this role, he oversees a comprehensive, integrative approach to holistic healthcare.

About the author

Raymond N Perrin DO PhD is a Registered Osteopath and Neuroscientist specialising in myalgic encephalomyelitis/chronic fatigue syndrome (ME/CFS). His present academic posts include Honorary Clinical Research Fellow at the School of Health Sciences in the Faculty of Biology, Medicine and Health at the University of Manchester, Manchester, UK and Honorary Senior Lecturer in the Allied Health Professions Research Unit, University of Central Lancashire, Preston, UK. He is also Research Director of the FORME Trust and Founder and Clinical Director of the Perrin Clinic™.

Treating a patient for backpain in 1989 led him to the concept that there was a structural basis to ME/CFS. He has spent over 35 years conducting clinical trials, researching the medical facts and sifting the scientific evidence while successfully treating an increasing number of ME/CFS, fibromyalgia and long COVID sufferers and teaching fellow osteopaths, chiropractors and physiotherapists the fundamentals of the Perrin Technique™.

For his service to osteopathy, Dr Perrin was appointed a vice-patron of the University College of Osteopathy (formerly the BSO) and in 2015 became the very first winner of the Research and Practice Award from the Institute of Osteopathy.

Introduction

Dear Reader,

This is a guidebook to aid practitioners in the treatment of long COVID and to help practitioners and sufferers to understand what is going wrong with their body and how they can help fight this complex, cruel disorder.

The theories and techniques explained in this book are all based on a doctorate, which I received after 11 years of clinical research into post-viral fatigue syndrome more commonly known as myalgic encephalomyelitis/chronic fatigue syndrome (ME/CFS) at the University of Salford, UK. What these theories and techniques are can be found in Chapter 4.

Since 2005, I have continued my post-Doc research at the University of Central Lancashire and the University of Manchester, UK. I have also been kept busy lecturing to the medical and scientific world on the lymphatic system of the brain and how it is disturbed in ME/CFS and fibromyalgia, plus teaching my techniques to those who wish to learn my approach. Since 2020 I have included long COVID in my work.

Teaching my theories wasn't easy in the beginning, as there was no proof that a lymphatic system of the brain even existed in the first place, never mind any problems with its drainage. Everything changed in 2012, when there was a breakthrough discovery at the University of Rochester in New York State.

Scientists, using a new type of brain scan, were able visually to show that the fluid in the brain did indeed drain into the lymphatics, and in 2015 a group from the University of Virginia discovered true lymphatic vessels lining the brain in mice. Finally, after so many years, the foundation of my main theory as to what was going wrong in patients with ME/CFS was being backed up by scientific discovery... albeit in rodents. It was then that I started writing the second edition of my first book – called simply *The Perrin Technique* - and during that writing process, further scans of human brains have revealed a major system of lymphatic drainage of the central nervous system which may, according to scientists around the world, provide a pathway that is affected in many neurological disorders, including long COVID. I developed the Perrin Technique™ in 1989 to improve this drainage system, so it is nice to know that finally science has caught up.

11 March 2020

Most of us won't forget this date. If your illness has affected your memory, and it often does, this was the day the World Health Organization's Director-General, Dr Tedros Adhanom Ghebreyesu, declared the novel coronavirus (COVID-19) outbreak a global pandemic. It was also the day of my 21st wedding anniversary. Most normal people don't spend their anniversary writing a letter to their research colleagues predicting long COVID. Fortunately, my wife Julie understood that I had to get the warning out there and so I wrote a letter to be published in a journal with my theories. This was aptly given the title by my research colleague, NHS consultant Dr Adrian Heald, 'Into the looking glass: Post-viral syndrome post COVID-19'.

My research colleagues and I warned the international medical community that in the aftermath of COVID-19 there would be millions around the world affected with what we christened 'Post COVID-19 syndrome'. The letter was subsequently published in June 2020 in the international scientific journal *Medical Hypotheses*.

Unfortunately, we were right about the conservative estimate. As I finish this book there are 65 million people worldwide with the syndrome, and probably millions of others left undiagnosed. Luckily for many, I had developed the Perrin Technique™ in 1989 to improve the lymphatic drainage system, so practitioners trained in this technique have been able to help thousands of long COVID sufferers around the world since the early days of the pandemic. Also on the plus side, there have been hundreds of scientists citing our paper in major international journals, with at least one new paper a week quoting our vision of the future we now know is all too real. Due to our work and the research of many others, the governments, scientists and health authorities around the world have started to seriously look into this disorder and other conditions such as ME/CFS as major neurological diseases.

For patients

In the Autumn of 2022 my publisher, Georgina, asked me to write a book on long COVID. Although much of this book is aimed at clinical and medical researchers and practitioners, some sections will hopefully guide you, the patient, along your own individual road to recovery:

- If you have long COVID and are unable to concentrate sufficiently to read long sections of text, the first section of Chapter 4 is for you, as it sums up my theory of diagnosis and treatment of this complex disorder.
- The Appendix on frequently asked questions also provides a quick guide to treatment.
- If you have a little more energy, then the self-massage and home exercise routines in Chapter 7 will be helpful and can also be viewed online in a step-by-step video guide available on YouTube and via the link at www.theperrintechnique.com.

However, you should not just rely on the self-massage and exercises in this book, though it is very important that you do these, as they will definitely help. It is always best to do the whole treatment programme under the direction of a qualified practitioner to confirm the diagnosis and to improve your outlook.

If you wish to start having treatment with the Perrin Technique™, please try to find a practitioner near to you who is a trained and a licensed Perrin Technique™ practitioner if possible. If there are none in your neighbourhood, seek out a practitioner trained and experienced in both cranial techniques and manual therapy. They should be able to follow the treatment instructions and be equipped to help you.

If your condition is more complicated, then a multidisciplinary approach including help by your Perrin Technique™ practitioner should be useful in even the most complex presentations.

I wish you every success with your treatment and progress to better health.

Ray Perrin
July 2024

Symptoms and body systems

I'll never know what happened, I was full of energy and life
Now I'm this drained carcass, Who's of no use to my wife
One day my 'joie de vivre', It just got up and left
So now I'm sitting here, feeling shattered and bereft
I battled with 'the virus', I should be lucky to be alive
But it's left me feeling guilty, With a bruised and dented pride

I try to rest whenever I can, and I try not to 'overdo'
But some jobs still need doing, but it's rare I'm tempted to
My poor old legs feel weak, as if they're made of lead
When I need to go upstairs, I have to lie down on the bed
My body just feels beaten, my muscles and joints all ache
But once I pop, I cannot stop, I hope you can relate?

My digestion too is failing, I'm bloating all the time
I hate to discuss my bowels, but find I do it all the time
Some days my heart beats faster, I fear I'm going to die
I try to sit down and be calm, I really, really try
They've sent me for appointments, had many scans and tests
But I just seem to baffle them, and the best of the NHS

They tell me it's 'long COVID', That in time I will recover
But getting through each day, It's getting hard to bother
All my energy has been depleted, It's not 'all in my head'
There's an army of people like me, 2 million or so I've read
I need to be a little kinder, to celebrate each small success
Pray the good times soon extend, and bad days get much less

©Dr Lisa Riste

Chapter 1

Long COVID: What's really going on?

'Poor Alice! It was as much as she could do, lying down on one side, to look through into the garden with one eye.'

Lewis Carroll

Alice's Adventures in Wonderland, p. 13

Case: Iain's story

At the end of January 2023 I burst into tears as I opened the front door of Perrin's Corner and stepped outside. Dr Perrin had just declared it to be 'D-Day'. I was finally discharged. What I hadn't been consciously aware of until the tears gave me away, was that I had spent a long time uncertain that I would ever be well again.

I caught COVID-19 in April 2020. I had a bit of a sore throat and a headache. I hadn't suffered any problems with taste, smell or breathing and felt that I had got off lightly. I was finding my daily duties of caring for my young adult daughter, who suffers with ME/CFS and fibromyalgia, increasingly difficult. I was spending more and more time either in bed or on the sofa. Another daughter couldn't manage to go to work and joined me on the sofa where, on a good day, I got to experience her favourite Netflix shows. On a bad day, even watching TV was too much for me. I couldn't cook, I could read very little, I couldn't go out and see anyone or run errands, even conversation was difficult. I would be knocked out for a few hours if I spoke to my parents on the phone. Eventually, my wife connected the dots and had a conversation with the man treating our youngest for ME. A trip to see Dr Raymond Perrin revealed that I had post-COVID fatigue, as did my eldest and middle daughters.

You may remember that shopping involved queueing and going one way around the shop and scrambling for toilet rolls … and I could be of no help whatsoever. My wife, Michelle, as well as working full time, had to deal with these extended domestic chores, doing all of the cooking and cleaning and massaging three of us every day. She would get up, work online, get our breakfast, go back into her office, stop to get us drinks, lunch, do the shopping, get dinner and then massage us all.

After a few months of being treated with the Perrin Technique™ in the clinic and at home I saw some improvement and could manage a short daily walk around the block. However, the progress was not in a straight line and I would plateau for several weeks at a time. It would be a joy to manage a few stretches and a longer walk, only to be unable to do them a few days later. I was constantly adjusting how long I thought it might take to get better and when I would be able to do more to support my family. My eldest and middle daughters were both back at work and discharged by Dr Perrin. I was still struggling physically, and the longer it went on, mentally.

Christmas came and went, with me doing next to nothing in the way of buying, wrapping, decorating and cooking.

A year after starting treatment, I remember being able to drive for a couple of hours, taking my daughter and son-in-law across country to a festival. I dropped them off and drove another half an hour to a quieter place to camp. I had to lie down for an hour before putting up my tent. I did nothing that evening. I did nothing the next day, I was so tired. By the time I arrived back to pick up my daughter from the festival, I had needed 48 hours rest for one 2½-hour drive. Despite how drained I felt, it was a huge milestone for me, to have driven for so long.

I have so many memories of sitting in various chairs and on benches, unable to complete a walk or a simple task. I promised some shelves for my now well daughter who had managed to get back to work and move out of home. I remember gathering some tools and wood together outside, then, unable to continue, sitting for a couple of hours in a garden chair before packing it all away again.

Dr Perrin and his colleagues, fellow Perrin Technique™ practitioners, were a continual support, encouraging me and advising little tweaks and changes I could make along the way to improve my recovery. A year after that exhausting 2½-hour drive, I was well enough to commit to lengthier drives and eventually, in August to October 2022, I helped two friends by driving a support vehicle across the USA, from Philadelphia to Phoenix, while they cycled from New York to Los Angeles. At the beginning of the ride, I would be careful to manage my energy and take rests throughout the day. Six weeks into the ride, I realised I was no longer doing this. At last, I was capable of an average day without wearing myself out.

As I write this in January 2024, a year after I was discharged, I am still hearing, all over the country, of people who have not yet 'got over' COVID-19, but suffer with various ailments, but particularly with exhaustion. As I tell my story I am met with fascination and surprise, and occasionally scepticism. Two of my daughters got long COVID and were better after a few months of the Perrin Technique™. It took me a lot longer, a full 2½ years, but I too am better, and I no longer have to concern myself with conserving energy or worry that I won't be able to manage something. For that I am grateful to Dr Raymond Perrin.

Iain Every, Ashton-under-Lyne, UK
Patient of Dr Raymond Perrin

The naming of the disease

I mentioned in the Introduction the paper 'Into the looking glass', which I wrote with colleagues at the beginning of the pandemic in 2020.[1] In this paper we named the disease 'Post-COVID-19 syndrome' as that was exactly what we predicted would happen, i.e. after patients had been hit with COVID-19, some would suffer from a long-term collection of symptoms (a syndrome).

According to a paper in October 2020 in the journal *Social Science and Medicine*[2] the terms 'long COVID' – and 'long-haul COVID' – were collectively used by patients themselves in the first months of the pandemic. Patients, many with initially 'mild' illness, used various kinds of evidence and advocacy to demonstrate a longer, more complex course of illness than that originally announced by authorities. 'Long COVID' could actually be the first illness named through patients finding one another on social media platforms. Through various media this name reached formal clinical and policy channels in just a few months, in September 2020, with the paper 'Long-haul COVID' in the journal *Neurology*.[3]

The rest, as they say, is history, with at present over 2500 peer-reviewed articles on long COVID published across all sections of medicine since 2020. The term 'long COVID' is not used by all. The purists in the medical world use the more scientific term 'post-acute sequelae SARS-CoV-2 infection' or 'PASC'.

Defining long COVID

The National Institute for Health Care Excellence (NICE) in the UK has classified the condition into two types:[4]

1. Ongoing symptomatic COVID-19 for people with symptoms continuing on for four to 12 weeks, and
2. Post-COVID-19 syndrome for people who still have symptoms for more than 12 weeks.

Long COVID patients have been classified by the International Classification for Diseases (ICD-10-CM) with a specific code: 'Post COVID-19 Condition, unspecified' (UO9.9)[5] and ICD-11 code (RA02).[6]

The World Health Organization (WHO) defines long COVID as:[7]

'a syndrome that occurs in individuals with a history of probable or confirmed SARS-CoV-2 infection, usually 3 months from the onset of COVID-19 with symptoms that last for at least 2 months and cannot be explained by an alternative diagnosis. Common symptoms include fatigue, shortness of breath and cognitive dysfunction but also others'.

The Centers for Disease Control and Prevention (CDC) in the US define it as 'new, persistent or evolving symptoms that are present four or more weeks after the initial infection'.[8]

But by far the simplest definition is stated in *The Long COVID Handbook* by Gez Medinger and Professor Danny Altman:

'long COVID is a long-term consequence of SARS-CoV-2 infection lasting beyond the initial 'acute' phase affecting multiple bodily organs and systems causing a huge variety of symptoms and of varying severity and duration, potentially relapsing and remitting over time'.[9]

The Office of National Statistics (ONS) in the UK estimated 1.9 million people living in private households in the UK (2.9% of the population) were already experiencing long COVID symptoms three years after the epidemic hit the UK (March 2023).[10]

Alas, at the time of writing this book, patients with long COVID suffer the same stigmas and barriers to proper healthcare as was, and still is, the case for many patients suffering from ME/CFS. The problem is that long COVID symptoms are difficult to distinguish from a wide range of other conditions (see Chapter 2 for a detailed discussion).

To try and address this issue, some questionnaires have been developed by clinical research scientists specifically for long COVID, such as the Symptom Burden Questionnaire™ for long COVID (SBQ™-LC) developed by Sarah Hughes and colleagues at the University of Birmingham. This is a patient-reported outcome measure examining a comprehensive list of most symptoms complained of affecting all organs and bodily systems.[11]

One of the leading researchers into diagnostic evaluation of ME/CFS is Professor Lenny Jason who, together with his colleagues at De Paul University in Chicago, has spent many years developing the internationally-recognised De Paul Questionnaire for ME/CFS and has been equally busy looking at ways of accurately classifying long COVID.[12]

However, as time goes on, many patients who have suffered long COVID symptoms for two or three years have developed more and more long-term symptoms which match those of patients with ME/CFS and which fulfil the international consensus criteria for ME/CFS.[13]

At just the time I was working on the final rewrites for this book, on 11 June 2024, the United States National Academies of Sciences, Engineering and

Medicine (NASEM) hosted a webinar which proposed a new definition for Long COVID. This followed a US government request that the National Academy of Medicine (NAM) convene a committee to examine and update existing US definitions based on the latest scientific evidence, testimony from medical and scientific professionals, and input from patients and the public. The NAM Committee was chaired by Physician Dr Harvey V Fineberg, who is a noted researcher in the field of health policy and emeritus Dean of the Harvard School of Public Health.

One of the members of the committee was the International Association of CFS/ME Vice President, Lily Chu, MD. I have had the pleasure of knowing Lily for over 15 years as a member of the Association and of presenting my research work at the IACFS/ME conferences since 2009.

The main highlights of the 2024 NASEM Long COVID definition[14]

The following is a summary of the key findings of the Committee:

- Long COVID (LC) is an infection-associated chronic condition (IACC) that occurs after SARS-CoV-2 infection and is present for at least three months as a continuous, relapsing and remitting, or progressive disease state that affects one or more organ systems.
- It manifests in multiple ways. A complete enumeration of possible signs, symptoms, and diagnosable conditions of LC would have hundreds of entries. Any organ system can be involved, and LC patients can present with:
  - single or multiple symptoms, such as: shortness of breath, cough, persistent fatigue, post exertional malaise, difficulty concentrating, memory changes, recurring headache, lightheadedness, fast heart rate, sleep disturbance, problems with taste or smell, bloating, constipation, and diarrhea.
  - single or multiple diagnosable conditions, such as: interstitial lung disease and hypoxemia, cardiovascular disease and arrhythmias, cognitive impairment, mood disorders, anxiety, migraine, stroke, blood

clots, chronic kidney disease, postural orthostatic tachycardia syndrome (POTS) and other forms of dysautonomia, myalgic encephalomyelitis/ chronic fatigue syndrome (ME/CFS), mast cell activation syndrome (MCAS), fibromyalgia, connective tissue diseases, hyperlipidemia, diabetes, and autoimmune disorders such as lupus, rheumatoid arthritis, and Sjogren's syndrome.

- Important features include:

  o It can follow asymptomatic, mild, or severe SARS-CoV-2 infection. Previous infections may have been recognized or unrecognized.

  o It can be continuous from the time of acute SARS-CoV-2 infection or can be delayed in onset for weeks or months following what had appeared to be full recovery from acute infection.

  o It can affect children and adults, regardless of health, disability or socioeconomic status, age, sex, gender, sexual orientation, race, ethnicity or geographic location.

  o It can exacerbate pre-existing health conditions or present as new conditions.

  o It can range from mild to severe. It can resolve over a period of months or can persist for months or years.

  o It can be diagnosed on clinical grounds. No biomarker currently available demonstrates conclusively the presence of LC.

  o It can impair individuals' ability to work, attend school, take care of family and care for themselves.

  o It can have a profound emotional and physical impact on patients and their families and caregivers.

How does long COVID affect the body?

Long COVID affects the communication between the internal organs and the musculoskeletal components of the body. This organ of communication is known as the **sympathetic nervous system** which may be likened to a transmission station in a power grid.

In our homes and at work, we use electricity for lighting, cooking, refrigerating and freezing, for electrical appliances, and for music centres, TVs and computers. The electrical energy required is produced by power stations and is monitored by controllers in transmission stations, which channel the amount of electricity through to us, the consumers.

If we were all suddenly to use substantially more electricity, simultaneously, the transmission station would allow more electricity to flow, signalling to the power stations to produce more energy. This occurs, for example, at half-time during major international televised sporting events, when everybody turns on the kettle at the same time to make a cup of tea.

If something were to go wrong with the operator, or the equipment in the transmission station were to develop a fault, the power required to cope with the increased demand would be insufficient. This would eventually lead to a power cut and blackout. Alternatively, if a situation were to arise when too much electricity passed into the household's supply, an overload or power surge could damage the appliances in use at that time.

In the body, the brain and the muscles are the principal 'electrical appliances', utilising most of the energy produced. The power station of the body is the gastrointestinal system (gut), together with the respiratory system, which consumes fuel in the form of food together with oxygen to produce the energy.

The sympathetic nervous system is the transmission station, which connects the visceral 'power station' of the body to the neuro-musculoskeletal 'appliance'.

To understand this more clearly, first here are a few facts that you need to know about the nervous system.

The nervous system can be divided into the central and peripheral systems. The central nervous system consists of the brain and the spinal cord, the peripheral system, which spreads out to the rest of the body, is further subdivided into the somatic and the autonomic nervous systems.

The somatic nervous system is associated with the voluntary control of body movements via motor nerves controlling the skeletal muscles plus sensory nerves receiving information from all over the body. The autonomic nervous system, on the other hand, regulates a variety of body processes that take place without conscious effort, as described in further detail in Chapter 2.

The autonomic nervous system is further divided into separate systems. The main one related to long COVID is the sympathetic nervous system, which makes the body ready for the 'fight or flight' response during any impending threat, as described on page 94. On the other hand, the parasympathetic nervous system inhibits the body from overworking and restores it to a calm and composed state and, until recently, was never thought to be a major factor in the disease process, unlike the sympathetic nerves. However, due to new findings, especially through the work of Dr Stephen Porges who in 1994 introduced his controversial 'polyvagal theory', we now know different. Dr Porges has discovered that there are not just two components to the autonomic nervous system, but in fact the main parasympathetic pathway is divided into two sections, front (ventral) and back (dorsal). The ventral vagus is a signalling system for motion, emotion and communication which forms our social engagement system; this is the part of the vagus nerve that is well known.[15]

The dorsal vagus in humans is a more recent discovery. It is a remnant of our primitive ancestry and is advanced in reptiles and possums, which use it when they play dead as a defence mechanism. It is the immobilisation system, which is our passive defence system and, if overstimulated, can lead to pathological mechanisms that cause symptoms such as bradycardia (extremely slow heart rate) and sleep apnoea, when some sufferers stop breathing for a dangerously long time in their sleep.

Many anatomists and scientists don't believe that the dorsal vagus exists in humans but I'm a fan of Dr Porges' work and I feel that both front (ventral) and back (dorsal) vagus nerves can be affected biomechanically by problems in the suboccipital region at the very top of the neck, and so this is an important region to examine and treat in some long COVID patients. Improving spinal movement and stability in this region between the top of the neck and the head can help balance the overall autonomic control.

The inflammatory reflex

The vagus nerve transmits signals from the body to the central nervous system when stimulated by cytokines (cell signalling chemicals), basically telling the brain that you are sick. Eighty per cent of these sensory vagal nerves have their nucleus in the brain stem. When peripheral cytokines stimulate the vagus there is a mirror response within the brain, leading to increased inflammatory cytokines being produced by the glial cells (explained on page 96).

Dr Kevin J Tracey, a neurosurgeon, and his team of scientists in Manhasset, New York, discovered that the vagus nerve, as well as conducting information from organs to the brain and back again, also modulates inflammation around the body, reducing the production of pro-inflammatory cytokines. Tracey showed that immune responses are controlled by autonomic reflex circuits similar to how the heart rate is controlled. He named this circuit the 'inflammatory reflex'.

Electrical implants that stimulate the vagus nerve have been used to treat conditions such as epilepsy. So, Tracey and his team used vagal nerve stimulators implanted through a small incision in the neck that turned off cytokine responses, improving symptoms of patients with rheumatoid arthritis by reducing the inflammation.[16]

The gateway reflex

There are also gateways in the spinal cord regulated by local sympathetic nerve activations that are stimulated by gravity. Pain, which increases the number of cytokines, attracts T-helper immune cells to the dorsal vessels, which pass into the central nervous system, through the blood–brain–barrier to infiltrate the central nervous system and trigger neuroinflammation.

This process is known as the 'gateway reflex' and is activated by stress, which acts on the paraventricular nucleus in the hypothalamus, leading to neuroinflammation in the brain. It has also been shown that, by electrically stimulating certain muscles, neuroinflammatory gateways are created at different levels of the spinal cord.[17]

A neuroscientist at Harvard University, Mike Van Elzakker, also believes neuroinflammation irritating autonomic control in the brainstem is a main part of the process leading to many neuroimmune disorders.[18] He classifies diseases similar to long COVID (such as ME/CFS) as auto-inflammatory disorders, where the crosstalk between the glial cells (see page 96) that surround the vagus nerve and the mast cells that produce inflammation-inducing chemicals such as cytokines, prostaglandins and the tumour necrosis factor-alpha (TNFα), further activate the vagus. This can lead to an auto-inflammatory condition when there is an ongoing inflammatory process without any pathogen to cause it (such as the corona virus that triggered the cytokine storm in the first place will have been long gone).

The vagus nerve also detects changes in the innate immune system that will occur whenever there is an infection causing a sickness response, such as a fever, helping to kill off viruses or bacteria that cannot survive at a higher body temperature.

What happens when the sympathetic nervous system breaks down?

When we are active, the sympathetic nervous system stimulates an increase of energy production and a release of stored energy. If this is not accomplished, the result is that the brain and muscles will not receive the nutrients normally obtained from the blood, and the natural function of the muscles, nerves and joints will break down. There will be a power cut in our body, and we will suffer fatigue.

This is precisely what occurs in patients suffering from long COVID. The body demands more energy, especially when under any form of stress, mental or physical. However, the mechanism which normally operates to transform the stored energy into a usable form is not functioning, and thus the patient's body simply stops working effectively.

It is therefore not surprising that in many cases long COVID is a profoundly debilitating disorder and requires as much rest as possible to reverse the process by minimising the amount of stress on the body. The power station analogy explains why some sufferers seem to display signs of too much sympathetic activity, such as palpitations and excessive sweating, as well as reduced sympathetic activity, such as fatigue and low blood pressure. The fault with the 'transmission station' could lead to the body working in overdrive as well as the power cut scenario, and sometimes in the same patient at the same time. Reducing the demand on the sympathetic nervous system helps the patient onto the road to a full recovery.

Conclusion

Long COVID is very similar to ME/CFS and FMS, all of which are due to a disturbance of the sympathetic nervous system which causes an imbalance of overall body functions leading to the many symptoms seen in these disorders. What happens next forms the basis of my 35 years' work in this field.

Just like Alice, when she went through the looking glass and found that everything was working upside down and back to front, as we pass through the looking glass of long COVID together, we will see that the sympathetic nervous system's control of the lymphatic system is disturbed, leading to a reversal of some of the lymphatic drainage of the brain, spinal cord and the rest of the body. This causes the neuro-inflammation and other effects of neurotoxicity that are affecting millions upon millions around the globe.

As you will see, knowing what happens through the looking glass has enabled me to develop aids to diagnosing and methods of treating long COVID, which all form part of the Perrin Technique™.

Chapter 2

Diagnosing long COVID

'I don't think they can hear me' she went on, as she put her head closer down 'and I'm nearly sure they can't see me. I feel somehow as if I were invisible.'

Lewis Carroll

Alice Through the Looking Glass and What Alice Found There, p. 89

Case: Kate's story

I contracted COVID-19 in March 2022 for the first time, during the Omicron wave. I'd been vaccinated and boosted, and at that point was a fit and active 48-year-old woman. My acute phase was mild, and I felt well enough after a few weeks to return to work and exercise. On a short, gentle run in early May I had the sensation of suddenly being out of energy and had to walk home. After that, my decline into the hell of long COVID was quick. In late May I had to take medical leave from my job as a university lecturer. My brain was unable to cope with work and I was increasingly fatigued. By the end of the summer, I was mostly housebound – a short walk would bring on post-exertional malaise, I felt

---

breathless, sleepless and in terrible back, neck and shoulder pain. I was experiencing unusual anxiety and low mood. At my sickest, I had to travel to the US for my father's funeral and a friend had to check me and my daughters in for our flights as my brain fog was too bad for me to do it.

Nobody knew much about long COVID, but I had friends with ME/CFS and I understood that's what it seemed like. The NHS was helpful up to a point, but the long COVID clinic was limited to managing symptoms and there seemed to be no known effective treatment. I felt very isolated. Caring for my kids as a single mother was overwhelmingly difficult, and I was scared about the future.

A friend told me about the Perrin Technique™, which he credited with curing his ME/CFS. Very luckily for me, Dr Perrin's clinic was a 20-minute drive away – even that was a challenge, but I dragged myself there. On that first visit in October 2022, my osteopath, Ian Trotter, found that I fitted the diagnostic criteria for ME/CFS and explained how the Perrin Technique™ could help. I committed to a regime of regular sessions at the clinic, daily rotation exercises and self-massage. I was told that if the treatment worked for me, I could expect something like full recovery in 18 months.

It's now December 2023 – 14 months later. Though my treatment is still ongoing, I feel like a different person. There are other things I've done alongside the Perrin treatment that have helped – breathwork, meditation, hormone treatment, rest and stress reduction – but the Perrin Technique™ has been fundamental and transformative. I went back to work on a phased return three months ago and am about to return to my full, in-person teaching schedule. I can do so many things that I was scared I wouldn't ever be able to do again: I can work a full day (with a few rest breaks), drive on the motorway, walk outside for about 45 minutes and swim slow lengths. I can do gentle rehabilitation exercises with a physical trainer without being wiped out afterwards. I can go out for drinks with friends, see concerts and plan holidays. My moods are more stable, and I have a more consistent baseline of energy to draw upon every day, though I still have to be mindful of my resources and not overtax myself. I don't feel like a sick person anymore. I feel like someone who is able to enjoy her life, with a few reasonable adaptations. I'm so happy with the progress I've made, and I feel hopeful about the future.

Kate Feld, Ramsbottom, UK.
Patient of osteopath and licensed Perrin Technique™ practitioner Ian Trotter

The symptoms of long COVID

It is generally agreed that long COVID is a serious chronic condition following infection with the COVID-19 virus, where symptoms persist for more than three months.[1]

According to the UK's National Health Service website information page, the most common ongoing symptoms are: 'Extreme tiredness (fatigue), feeling short of breath, problems with memory and concentration ('brain fog'), heart palpitations, dizziness, joint pain and muscle aches'. Before we look at how the condition becomes chronic, let's look at all these, and other symptoms mentioned in the NHS list, in the light of what we know about the underlying problem here – dysfunctional lymphatic drainage from the central nervous system.

Once you have read this book, long COVID and its symptoms should no longer be a mystery. By understanding the mechanisms that cause this disorder (see Chapter 4) one can logically explain all the varied symptoms that patients suffer. Over the past four years, many patients have asked me whether a particular symptom could be due to their long COVID; I have gone through the NHS list to try to answer those questions.

I say 'could be due to long COVID' because, of course, there is always a possibility of a comorbidity (additional condition) being present. In other words, the patient could be suffering from more than one condition and the symptom may be due to a completely different disease as well as long COVID. Any new complaint should always be thoroughly investigated to rule out any serious pathology, and there are plenty of comorbidities that require their own specific treatment approach. As a general rule I would suspect the onset of a different disease if new symptoms seem to begin out of the blue and gradually worsen, when the major symptoms of the long COVID are responding well to treatment.

Fatigue: The fatigue in long COVID is typically both physical and mental and is aggravated by exertion and not relieved by rest. The lymphatic system should drain away excess lactic acid created by exertion; however, in long COVID, neurotoxins affect the central autonomic control in the brain which disturbs the sympathetic nerve control of lymphatic vessels. This leads to a retrograde flow of lymph, resulting in a raised level of lactic acid following low-level exercise, plus a reduced clearance after exercise. The mental fatigue associated with long COVID is due partly to altered blood flow to parts of the brain resulting from sympathetic nerve dysfunction and partly to disturbed neurotransmission within the brain due to neurotoxic overload caused by backflow of the neuro-lymphatic system (see Brain fog, page 19, opposite).

Feeling short of breath (also known as dyspnoea or dyspnea): Breathlessness is a common symptom in long COVID due to the Coronavirus inhaled by the lungs leading to severe acute respiratory syndrome (SARS). COVID-19 was originally known as SARS II. Apart from the obvious effect on the lungs, the autonomic dysfunction that occurs will lead to disturbance in the control of the cardiovascular system and ventilation.

Brain fog: One of the most common symptoms of long COVID is described by many patients as 'brain fog' or, as I like to call it, 'muzziness'. Their ability to think properly about anything is usually disturbed. The main parts of the brain affected by neurolymphatic drainage problems are the frontal and prefrontal lobes concerned with thought, plus the basal ganglia and thalamus, which are concerned with emotion and relay messages from the frontal region to all over the brain. This leads to the brain fog that some patients find the worst of all the symptoms, especially if prior to their illness they had a job that required major cognitive skills. Owing to the connection with the limbic system, it makes them even more depressed.

Palpitations: Many patients with long COVID have noticeable rapid, strong, or irregular heartbeats that are aggravated by exertion or stress. The palpitations are caused by the build-up of neurotoxicity in the brain (see Chapter 3) leading to disturbance in the sympathetic and parasympathetic nervous control of the heart via the cardiac plexus, which is situated at the base of the heart. In fact, the link made between long COVID and the autonomic control of the heart goes back to the American Civil War, when the condition was known as 'irritable heart disease' or 'soldier's heart'.

Dizziness (also termed vertigo): Dizziness can be due to problems in the brain, blood flow to the head and/or a disturbance in the vestibular apparatus, the balance mechanism within the ear. In long COVID, there is a toxic overload in the central nervous system affecting the brain, plus there is a disturbance of the autonomic control of the cerebral circulation and, to make matters even worse, one of the main pathways of the neurolymphatic drainage system is the perivascular space of the blood vessels supplying the eighth cranial nerve, the vestibulocochlear, which controls balance. A build-up of toxins when there is a backflow of this drainage leads to dizziness.

Arthralgia (joint pain): Arthralgia is usually present in many areas of the body in patients with long COVID. The pain is due to two factors: (i) the areas controlling pain in the thalamus and basal ganglia of the brain have become dysfunctional due to neurotoxins, exacerbating pain throughout the body; and (ii) disturbed sympathetic nerves affecting sensory nerves and local nociceptors (pain receptors) in the joints. The joints become painful but not swollen unlike in arthritis. Long COVID is not arthritic disease, so if the joints of the patient are swollen then joint pain is due to another condition, possibly SLE (lupus) or rheumatoid arthritis. Sometimes the patient will complain of swollen hands or feet, but this is usually due to oedematous changes resulting from problems with their lymphatic drainage and not arthritis.

Myalgia (muscular pain): Myalgia is nearly always present in patients with long COVID, but not usually as widespread as with the condition fibromyalgia. Clinically I find most of the pain is in the upper trunk and the limbs, aggravated by exertion. The pain is due to three factors: (i) the control areas of pain in the thalamus and basal ganglia of the brain have become dysfunctional due to neurotoxins exacerbating pain throughout the body; (ii) disturbed sympathetic nerves affecting sensory nerves and local nociceptors (pain receptors) in the muscles and tendons. This disturbance of sympathetic nerve activity can reduce blood flow in the muscles. The resultant ischaemia further irritates the nociceptors, leading to worsening pain; and (iii) increased lactic acid can also cause myalgia.

Those are listed as the key symptoms, but the NHS website goes on to say that there are lots of additional post-COVID symptoms, including:

Anosmia (loss of smell): This has been a common symptom in the COVID-19 outbreak and may continue long after the initial infection has passed. The pro-inflammatory cytokines produced by the immune system become congested within the perivascular lymphatic drainage through the olfactory pathway in the perforations of the cribriform plate, part of the ethmoid bone lying above the nasal cavity. As explained on page 72, this has been shown to be the main neurolymphatic drainage point in the cranium. The increased toxicity and inflammation will result in damage to the olfactory nerves, leading to a disturbed sense of smell and, in some extreme cases, total loss of smell.

Anxiety (not primary, but secondary to the disease): This is a very common symptom in long COVID. The limbic system in the brain controls the emotions and is the main region targeted by neurotoxins when there is a backflow and congestion of the neurolymphatic system. This is compounded by the stress caused by the condition and the worry that the symptoms will worsen if the patient exerts him/herself. The resultant inactivity in severe cases aggravates the anxiety state.

Chest pain or tightness: As described on page 31–32, in nearly all long COVID patients, whether male or female, there is a tender area in the upper lateral region of the breast tissue, roughly 2 cm superior and lateral to the left nipple. This is due to a confluence of two sensory nerve networks irritated by sympathetic nerve pathways from the thoracic duct and the cardiac plexus. Since the 1990s I have felt the sensitive region now known as Perrin's Point, together with congested lymph vessels in the breast tissue which can further lead to chest pain, in nearly all the thousands of ME/CFS patients I have examined and I am seeing the same in long COVID patients.

Cough: A persistent cough that may or may not be dry is a symptom of long COVID and is usually a result of sensitivities or allergies that are more common in this condition, with MCAS being a common comorbidity as explained in Chapter 9. Sometimes patients experience post-nasal drip when excess mucus drains down the throat, causing coughing, especially if it contains neurotoxins. Occasionally, in some patients I have seen irritation of the nerves supplying the diaphragm and intercostal muscles, leading to a chronic cough. Both breathlessness and coughs may persist due to the reversal of lymphatic drainage leading to increased fibroblast deposits producing fibrosis in the lungs, which is a very common finding in many long COVID patients.

Depression: The limbic system in the brain has been shown to be the most affected part of the brain when there is a restriction or backflow of the neurolymphatic system. This leads to most patients suffering from symptoms of depression. However, there is another major secondary cause of depression in long COVID. My name for this is TPOS ('thoroughly p****d off syndrome'!) and it is usually brought about by frustration – not being able to do any activity without suffering and not having any real proof of the illness, with many getting worse and becoming less active, which only aggravates their depression. It is a sad fact that most long COVID patients never receive 'get well' cards, as even their closest friends and family do not really understand why they are so ill, which leads to further frustration and depression.

Diarrhoea and/or constipation: These symptoms can be due to irritable bowel syndrome, which is a very common complaint among my long COVID patients as in gut dysbiosis (unbalanced gut microbiome). The autonomic nerve disturbance in long COVID can also lead to overstimulation or understimulation of bowel movements and resultant diarrhoea/constitpation and abdominal pain.

Headache: This is one of the most frequent symptoms of long COVID. It can be similar to migraine headache and is often due to the increase or decrease of blood flow in the head due to autonomic nervous system dysfunction. Congested toxins in the cranium outside of the brain can stimulate nociceptors (pain receptors) that can lead to severe piercing headaches, especially in the region of the forehead. Due to metabolic changes, patients may often be dehydrated or hypoglycaemic (low blood sugar), both common causes of headaches in long COVID. With a backflow of cerebrospinal fluid drainage, some symptoms such as headaches and nausea may be due to a very slight increase in intracranial pressure known as idiopathic intracranial hypertension.

Insomnia: Sleep disturbance in long COVID usually takes the form of insomnia that includes difficulty getting to sleep or waking throughout the night; however, sometimes it involves too much sleep (hypersomnia). Sleep is controlled in the brain in areas specifically targeted by toxins, such as the hypothalamus, pineal gland, thalamus and locus coeruleus; consequently, sleep/awake patterns and the quality of the sleep are affected.

Loss of appetite: Just as in ME/CFS, the severity of the symptoms may be due to a link with the hormone leptin. Leptin is released from fat cells to regulate energy balance by inhibiting hunger via signals to the brain, especially the hypothalamus, and if disturbed leads to neurotoxic damage of the fatty glial cells in the brain. This leads to increase or decrease in feelings of satiety, thereby affecting the appetite of the patient and can in some cases also lead to major cravings.

Nausea: In long COVID the toxic overload of the brain due to disturbed neurolymphatic drainage can lead to symptoms such as nausea when the patient is upright. In other words, this is an aspect of orthostatic intolerance (see page 57).The vestibular pathway in the ear may also be affected, leading to dizziness and nausea. Any toxic overload and disturbed autonomic control of the liver and gastrointestinal system can also lead to nausea.

Pins-and-needles/tingling in the skin (paraesthesia): Some patients with long COVID will complain of many unusual sensory symptoms, including pins-and-needles, often in different parts of their body. This is due to over-activity of the sympathetic nervous system due to neurotoxicity in the brain. Superficial sympathetic nerves lie adjacent to somatic sensory nerves and so near the skin surface there can be a crossover of neurological activity passing between the two nerves in what are known as ephapses (see page 32). This leads to these sensory disturbances which don't seem to follow the dermatomes – the normal distribution of areas of skin supplied by the specific sensory nerves.

Skin rashes and spots: Many patients with long COVID develop rashes and spots on the skin, mostly on the face, upper back and/or chest, but they can be anywhere on the body. These can be atopic skin reactions such as eczema and can also be caused by reactions to, or side effects of, some medicines commonly prescribed, but they are more commonly due to toxic overload affecting the control of the superficial lymphatic system which can cause many types of skin eruptions, such as acne and rosacea. Rosacea is an inflammatory chronic skin condition often seen in long COVID, leading to redness and raised spots. It is similar to acne and usually found on the face but can appear in all other parts of the body. It can be triggered by stress but has been linked mainly to types of pro-inflammatory and environmental toxins.

Sore throat: The post-nasal drip often complained of by long COVID patients is due to toxins draining from the inflamed nasal mucous membranes down to the throat. The neuroimmune system is compromised in long COVID, leading to lymphatic congestion in the neck; this in turn leads to the build-up of post-infectious toxins that can cause sore throats. Some patients with long COVID suffer from sore throats as part of chronic co-infections such as coxsackie-B and human herpes viruses, or chronic bacterial illnesses, such as borreliosis (Lyme disease).

Tinnitus: One of the main pathways of neurolymphatic drainage is the perivascular space of the blood vessels supplying the eighth cranial nerve, the vestibulo-cochlear nerve, which controls hearing. A build-up of toxins due to a backflow of lymphatic drainage in long COVID can lead to continuous buzzing or ringing in the ears as well as earache and other associated symptoms.

The development of long COVID

With careful consideration of 35 years of clinical experience and research findings in the field of ME/CFS (which is often a post-viral fatigue syndrome), I have established a theoretical model to explain how the signs and symptoms of long COVID develop (see Table 2.1).

This Table reflects the clinical history of all the long COVID patients I have seen since the spring of 2020.

Table 2.1: The stages of development leading to long COVID

Stage 1	Patients with long COVID all seem to have a predisposing history of sympathetic nervous system overload.
a	Physically – by being an overachiever at work, during study, or in sports. Rarely, it may be the opposite by being too sedentary.
b	Chemically – by constant exposure to environmental pollution.
c	Immunologically – by chronic infections or hypersensitivities to multiple allergens.
d	Psychologically/emotionally – by family and/or work-related mental stress.
Stage 2	In Stage 2 either a or b can occur before the other or they can occur concurrently, depending on the causes of the restricted flow of lymphatic drainage in the head and spine.
a	Lymphatic drainage from the brain shows signs of being impaired, mostly in the cribriform plate region of the ethmoid bone above the nasal passages, the neural pathways along the optic nerve behind the eye, the trigeminal pathways in the region of the upper jaw and the drainage along auditory pathways.
b	Lymphatic drainage of the central nervous system is also subject to disturbances in the spine, usually in the cervical or thoracic region, due to either a congenital, hereditary or postural defect and/or prior trauma.
Stage 3	Toxic effects due to the long-term dysfunction of central nervous system drainage will compound the chronic hyperactivity of the sympathetic nervous system; this further overloads the hypothalamus and subsequently, the sympathetic nervous system.
Stage 4	The final trigger factor strikes – a SARS-CoV-2 (COVID-19) infection.

Stage 5	There will be a further disturbance in autonomic, as well as hormonal, function due to COVID-19, the spike protein of the virus, cytokines and other pro-inflammatory toxins enter the brain and directly affect control of the hypothalamus. Hormonal transport within the cerebrospinal fluid may be directly affected by this toxic overload. Further central neuro-inflammation due to disturbance of the vagal inflammatory reflex as a result of stress activating the hypothalamus and other peripheral spinal pathways of the gateway reflex.
Stage 6	Dysfunction of sympathetic control of the lymphatics, especially the thoracic duct, leads to a reflux of in the resultant retrograde lymph flow, causing varicose lymphatic vessels (see Figs 4, 5 and 6, pp. 34, 35, 36) predominantly in the neck, chest and abdomen. This also further reduces flow of cerebrospinal fluid into the lymphatics. The reversal of lymph leads to a build-up of large molecules in the body, especially the complement of proteins, leading to chronic autoimmune inflammatory response and increase in clotting factors in blood. Lymphatic drainage is also reversed in muscles leading to a build-up of T-lymphocytes and lactic acid, leading in turn to damage of muscle tissue and worsening fatigue. This also explains the build-up of fibroblastic activity due to backflow of lymph, that should drain away fibroblasts, leading to fibrosis of muscles and other tissues and organs in the body.
Stage 7	Further backflow of toxic drainage into the central nervous system, due to the retrograde lymphatics, results in increased neuro-inflammation and hypothalamic dysfunction and an even greater disturbance of lymphatic drainage.
Stage 8	The continuing irritation of the autonomic nervous system results in further systemic disturbances, leading to the chronic adaptive post-viral state known as long COVID.

The physical signs of long COVID

I once had the pleasure of hearing a Stanford Professor of Medicine, Dr Abraham Verghese, at an international ME/CFS conference in California when he made the most profound statement: 'The doctor's round … has become square'. In other words, instead of physically examining the patient, as in days gone by, most physicians are busy looking at a screen for pathological tests etc. In most cases, they should also be looking at and listening to the patient to work out what is really going on. As a trained osteopath, I listen to, observe and palpate all patients before making any diagnosis. Sometimes pathological tests and computers are needed to confirm the diagnosis, but one should always carry out a physical examination first. Although awareness of long COVID is much greater than in the early days of ME/CFS, many patients who suffer from long COVID are still left untreated, with the physician hoping that the patient will spontaneously recover, learn to live with the problem, or change doctors. Despite many, many scientific papers being published which demonstrate that long COVID is a real physical disease, with many different pathological findings, there are still many GPs who refuse to believe in a physical source of the symptoms and refer their patients to a psychiatrist.

In fact, many research papers have shown that neurological disorders are related to SARS-CoV-2, and can involve both the central nervous system and the peripheral nervous system. According to recent studies, more than a third of patients present neurological symptoms during the infection, and post-infectious symptoms often continue in the disease we now call long COVID.[2]

Although many in the medical profession now recognise long COVID and realise that there is something physically wrong with the patient, they do not know how to diagnose or how to treat it. Some of my patients who suffer from severe symptoms of long COVID have been to neurologists, undergone brain scans, X-rays, blood tests and many other exhaustive examinations, all of which have yielded inconclusive evidence that there is anything wrong at all besides possibly, in some cases, the finding of fibrotic tissue in one or more organs. Mostly the patient is told to get on with life as best they can and to try and forget about their symptoms. The usual advice given to sufferers is to rest until the body sorts itself out, or worse, to increase activity, which often causes the patient's symptoms to quickly deteriorate.

Sadly, many patients are just existing with long COVID, waiting for the miracle cure that never comes. Even more depressing is that often the patient's own family and friends do not give the patient the support they need. Even in cases where the patient does have a loving and caring family and group of friends, there is a lack of understanding regarding long COVID. This lack of understanding is compounded by some sections of the media, who often belittle the symptoms as just 'in the mind' and suggests that these patients are actually not that ill. How many 'get well' cards are ever received by long COVID patients? … Usually none!

The concept of the cause of long COVID being primarily biophysical rather than immunological is foreign to most of the medical profession. However, many doctors recognise that long COVID patients have physical signs and symptoms (see Fig. 1).

Fig. 1 shows the following five regions of tenderness or dysfunction have been identified in most of the long COVID sufferers that I have seen in the past three years:

1. Longstanding thoracic (upper back) spinal problems.
2. Varicose lymphatics.
3. Tenderness in the left breast at a point now referred to as Perrin's Point.
4. Tenderness in an area at the upper mid-section of the abdomen known as the coeliac or solar plexus.
5. Disturbance of the cranial rhythmic impulse (cranio-sacral rhythm).

1. Longstanding thoracic spinal problems (often with flatness, redness, heat or pain in mid-thoracic spine)

2. Varicose lymphatics

3. Perrin's point

4. Coeliac plexus (solar plexus) tendernes

5. Abnormal cranio-sacral rhythm (cranial rhythmic impulse)

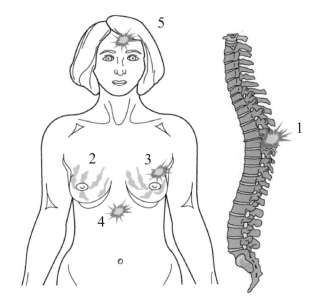

Fig. I The palpable and observable physical signs of long COVID.

Thoracic (upper back) spinal problems

As in ME/CFS, a prevailing observation in the clinical findings of long COVID is a mechanical disorder of the thoracic spine.

There is much truth in the famous song *Dry Bones* by the Delta Rhythm Boys. You know, the one which has the immortal lines:

'Your toe bone connected to your foot bone...'

'Your foot bone connected to your heel bone...'

and so on and so on until we get to the top of the body ...

'Your back bone connected to your shoulder bone...'

'Your shoulder bone connected to your neck bone...'

'Your neck bone connected to your head bone...'

'I hear the word of the Lord.'

What this song reminds us of is that any physical (genetic or otherwise) defect in one part of the body can have a major influence on another section. For instance, if one has one leg slightly shorter than the other it will lead to a compensatory lateral shift in the spinal column causing possible drainage problems in the spinal perivascular pathways and extra strain on the surrounding soft tissue, which includes the muscles, ligaments and fascia. This can then create extra pressure on the blood and lymph vessel walls, causing disturbed circulation and drainage. Likewise, an upper spinal problem can create a disparity in the forces placed on the legs and feet. This actually happened in clinic when a girl came in wearing callipers on her left lower leg. This was due to a weakness in her left ankle that for years had baffled her doctors. I discovered an upper spinal scoliosis (side-bending) that placed too much pressure on her left side, leading to eventual pain in the left leg, foot and ankle. Over the years she had compensated for the pain by using her right dominant side much more, resulting in the eventual weakness in her left ankle and foot requiring support.

Long-standing thoracic spinal problems

The most common structural disturbance that I have seen in long COVID patients is a flattening of the curvature in the mid-thoracic spine, usually accompanied by the presence of a kyphotic dorso-lumbar area (an abnormally exaggerated convex curvature in the lower back). An example of this defect is shown in Fig. 2(a) which can be compared with the healthy posture shown in Fig. 2(b). This postural defect is often caused by a prior condition, spinal osteochondrosis, also known as Scheuermann's disease, which affects spinal development in adolescence, and which may have occurred years before the onset of the characteristic symptoms of long COVID.

Also, when one feels the skin lying over the thoracic spine, it is usually hotter (but not always) than other regions of the trunk, which may indicate an underlying area of inflammation. Another common finding in this region in long COVID is the presence of trophic changes – that is, changes due to interruption of the nerve supply which affects nerve interactions with other cells, such as the skin, leading to molecular changes, including dryness, spots and rashes. Scars are also sometimes seen, indicating previous injury or surgery in the region. Also, abnormal amounts of redness in the skin overlying this region of the back are often seen after it is stimulated by a rubbing/stroking motion.

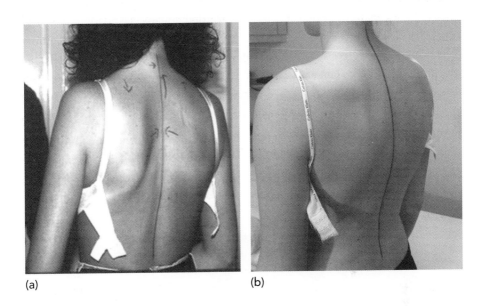

(a)   (b)

Fig. 2 Comparative photographs showing a flattened mid-thoracic spine. Photo (a) shows the familiar flattening of the mid-thoracic spine seen in many long COVID patients. This differs from a normal spinal posture in the healthy subject, photo (b).

Varicose lymphatics and Perrin's Point

In nearly all long COVID patients, whether male or female, there is a tender area in the upper lateral region of the breast tissue, roughly 2 cm superior and lateral to the left nipple (see Fig. 1 (marked with a '3') and Fig. 3 (marked with a 'X'). This finding is significant because the tender area almost always lies on the left side and is level with the position at which the thoracic duct turns to the left. The heart and the main blood vessels are supplied with sympathetic nerves via a bundle of nerves called the cardiac plexus, which has a greater concentration of nerves on the left than the right. Sympathetic nerves that are close to the skin run alongside the larger nerves that control movement and sensation in the body (the somatic nerves). Impulses cross over from sympathetic nerves to somatic sensory nerves and vice versa between the adjacent parallel nerve fibres via what are called ephapses.[3]

When the cardiac plexus is affected in long COVID, the sympathetic nerves send messages to the sensory nerves on the left side of the chest. The thoracic duct travels from the right side to the left side of body above the level of the nipple and so sympathetic nerves controlling the thoracic duct's pumping action are more on the left-hand side above the nipple line. Thus, when these nerves are irritated, they also disturb the adjacent sensory nerves. The resultant pain is at the confluence of these two networks of irritated sensory nerves. This tender spot is now known as 'Perrin's Point' (see the 'X' in Fig. 3).

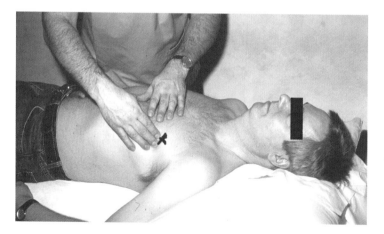

Fig. 3 Examining a male patient for 'Perrin's Point'. Gentle pressure at a point slightly superior and lateral to the left nipple, 'Perrin's Point'(X). The amount of sensitivity at this point appears to correspond to the severity of lymphatic engorgement in the breast tissue and also seems to mirror the gravity of the other symptoms.

Since the 1990s I have felt the sensitive region now known as Perrin's Point, together with congested lymph vessels in the cervical (neck) region and breast tissue, in nearly all of the thousands of ME/CFS patients I have examined. I am seeing the same in long COVID patients. The consistency of these lymphatics can best be described as a 'string of beads' and similar to varicose veins in the leg. Varicosities have been described before in the lymphatic system.[4, 5, 6] Large incompetent varicose lymphatics, known as 'megalymphatics', have often been seen when there is a backflow of fluid within the lymphatic vessels, due to a disturbance of the normal pumping mechanism. However, varicosities in the lymphatics are rarely discussed in clinics, due to the misconception that lymph flow can only be unidirectional due to a system of valves in the lymphatic vessels. Sluggish lymph flow is known to exist in many disease states and is treated by many practitioners worldwide who are trained in manual lymphatic drainage.[7]

However, the concept of a reverse pump causing an actual backflow is not generally recognised clinically. Thus, the possibility of a varicose lymph vessel is rarely considered when a GP or hospital consultant conducts an examination. Downward pressure due to thoracic duct pump dysfunction caused by sympathetic disequilibrium may lead to a contra-flow within the lymphatics,[8] damaging the valves and creating a pooling of lymphatic fluid with exaggerated 'beading' of the vessels. Stasis (fluid not moving) in these varicose lymphatic vessels creates a risk of toxic overload together with additional damage to the lymphatics and surrounding tissue.

Reflux of toxins via lymphatic vessels back into the cerebrospinal fluid will further irritate the central nervous system. Increased toxicity within the central nervous system continues to overload the sympathetic nerves, resulting in a downward spiral of deteriorating health.

From the earliest days of osteopathy, the importance of good lymphatic drainage in the thoracic duct has been seen as paramount to sustain health.[9, 10, 11, 12] It was emphasised that, together with good blood supply, it was equally important to have perfect drainage. This is the pathway I believe to be compromised mechanically as part of the root cause of people developing long COVID. Mechanical dysfunction such as this can be detected by palpation with the fingertips and can be released by gentle pressure and massage techniques applied to the cranium and the spine and surrounding soft tissue.

The healthy lymphatic vessel allows only unidirectional flow due to the system of valves illustrated in Fig. 4.

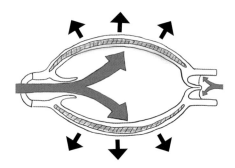

Fig. 4 Schematic illustration showing normal flow within a healthy lymphatic vessel. The valves in this healthy vessel are intact, preventing any backflow, thus maintaining a healthy, unidirectional drainage (note the smooth muscular wall of the lymphangion regulated by sympathetic nerves).

In long COVID, long before the person is infected by the coronavirus, retrograde flow of the lymphatics is produced by the reverse peristaltic wave of the thoracic duct that arises from dysfunctional sympathetic control of the duct's smooth muscle wall. This causes a reflux of fluid throughout the lymphatic system affecting individual lymph-collecting vessels (lymphangia), leading to the formation of varicose megalymphatics, initially in the neck and chest, as seen in Fig. 5 (a–c). Eventually, the lymphatic reflux causes damage to the valves and allows pooling of fluid in between them (Fig. 5 (b)). This leads to distension of the vessel wall with the characteristic enlarged beaded appearance of a varicose vessel as illustrated in Fig. 5 (c).

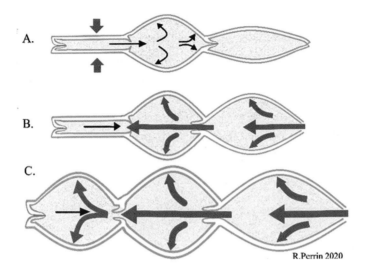

Fig. 5 The development of varicose megalymphatics: (a) The normal lymph flow before the illness. (b) Reversal of the central lymphatic pump forces the colourless lymph fluid back, damaging the valves that separate the adjacent collecting vessels (lymphangia). (c) The lymphangia expand due to the pressure and volume of the backward flowing lymph. This leads to the large, beaded vessels (varicose megalymphatics) palpated (felt with the fingertips) just beneath the skin in the chest of most long COVID patients.

Fig. 6/Plate 1 shows the top right section of the chest of a 61-year-old man. One can see the swollen, tortuous beaded vessels just beneath the collar bone adjacent to the right shoulder. This man suffered severely from ME/CFS for four years before being successfully treated with a two-year course of the Perrin Technique™ (see Chapter 4). The beaded appearance in Fig. 6/Plate 1 is due to damaged valves and subsequent retrograde flow and pooling of lymphatic fluid. This is similar to the formation of varicose veins, although it lacks the darker, bluish hue of superficial varicose veins. The fluid in the lymphatic vessel, known simply as 'lymph', is colourless and so these vessels are definitely lymphatic, and not blood vessels as they have the same colour as the overlying skin.

These vessels also have a much larger diameter (around 5 mm) than do healthy superficial lymphatic vessels (around 0.5 mm), which are normally extremely difficult to palpate, never mind actually see with the naked eye. It is extremely rare to see such pronounced superficial varicose megalymphatics as illustrated here. However, I have been able to feel the presence of varicose lymphatic vessels in the chests of virtually all the ME/CFS and FMS patients I have seen since 1989 and over the past four years, since the first long COVID case was treated in my clinic, I have felt these varicose megalymphatics in all my long COVID patients.

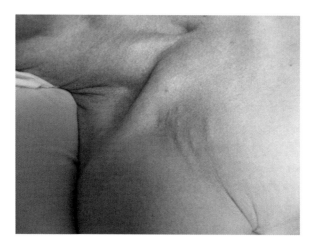

Fig. 6 Right subclavicular varicose megalymphatics, lacking the bluish hue of varicose veins, in a patient with ME/CFS (see also Plate 1).

Fig. 7/Plate 2 is a photo taken by licensed Perrin Technique™ practitioner Ian Trotter showing multiple varicose megalymphatics seen throughout the left breast of a 73-year-old patient with long COVID.

Tenderness at the coeliac or solar plexus

The largest major plexus of the autonomic nervous system, uniting two large coeliac ganglia, is known as the **coeliac plexus**, more commonly referred to as the 'solar plexus' (see Fig. 1).

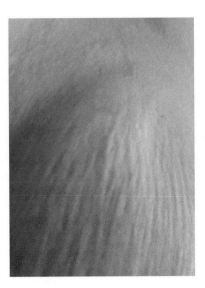

Fig. 7. Megalymphatics throughout the left breast of a 73-year-old long COVID patient (see also Plate 2).

Through its connections, the solar plexus is excellent as an indicator for any visceral disturbances from the waist down. Tenderness in this abdominal region, known as the epigastrium, seems to be directly related to the severity of any lower extremity fatigue and/or abdominal problem. This, as with Perrin's Point, is due to impulses passing across the 'ephapses' – connections between adjacent sensory and sympathetic nerves – and, again, is usually much more tender in long COVID patients.

On palpation, the epigastrium is also usually warmer than the rest of the abdomen, possibly due to the back flow of inflammatory toxins pumping down the thoracic duct into the upper regions of the abdomen and also the build-up of neurogenic inflammation from coeliac plexus overload.

Disturbance in the cranio-sacral rhythm

There is a palpable rhythmic pulsation along the spinal cord and around the brain, together with that of normal breathing, which is transmitted to the rest of the body and is termed the 'cranial rhythmic impulse' (CRI) or the 'cranio-sacral rhythm'. The rhythm is also known by some osteopaths as the 'involuntary mechanism' and by others as the 'primary respiration' as it is believed by some to be the inherent driver of all other mechanisms and rhythms in the body. Most of the osteopathic profession believe this pulse to be a movement through the tension and continuity of membranes and fascia. The fascia is the name for connective tissue throughout the body containing many lymphatic vessels that is continuous with the membranes that surround the brain and spinal cord, the meninges, thus allowing the different motions, and tensions, of the body to be transmitted everywhere.

William Garner Sutherland (1873–1954), the founder of cranial osteopathy, proposed that there was a primary respiratory mechanism created within the central nervous system and via the spinal cord, with the bones in the cranium all moving in a rhythmic pattern together with the sacrum at the base of the spine.[11]

Sutherland proposed that the primary respiratory mechanism produces a rhythmic alternation of flexion and extension of structures in the midline. This movement occurs simultaneously with rhythmic external and internal rotation of all paired lateral structures.[12]

Lymphatic vessels with muscular walls that expand and contract exist throughout the body, which creates a powerful pumping mechanism.[4]

It has been shown that the thoracic duct pump influences the drainage of CSF/lymph from the central nervous system. Together with the pulse rate and the effects of breathing, a separate underlying rhythm may be induced which is very possibly the aforementioned 'involuntary mechanism'. This rhythm echoes along the lymphatic system, resonating throughout the entire body, and can be palpated (felt) by trained practitioners. In long COVID patients it is often slower, arrhythmic, plus its intensity is shallower than in healthy people, and in very severe cases it is almost absent. A disturbed CRI was found in all the long COVID patients that I have examined clinically and during my research.

My theory is that the CRI is produced by the drainage of cerebrospinal fluid (CSF) from the brain and spine into the lymphatics. It is a product of the two dynamic fluid systems, each with its own distinct rhythm, coming together to produce this third cranial rhythm, similar to a large incoming wave on a beach colliding with a much shallower wave going out, creating a third wave.[13]

My theory is also supported by the fact that CSF drainage into the lymphatics, the glymphatic system, in humans has now been proven to exist and that neuroscientists have shown that breathing and posture affect the movement of CSF and thus aid CSF drainage to the lymphatics.[14]

The two minor physical signs

Over the years I have observed two other notable signs that appear in many cases, but they are not present in the majority, so I call them the minor physical signs. These are stretch marks and pupil dilation.

- **Stretch marks**, known medically as 'striae', are caused by damaged collagen fibres close to the skin surface. Striae are often seen on the thighs and breast tissue of long COVID patients and are most probably due to damage to collagenous anchoring ligaments attached to surface lymphatic vessels. This could occur when there is a major backflow of lymph and is seen in many long COVID patients who have never been obese or pregnant, which are the two most common physiological causes of striae.
- **Pupil dilation**. In long COVID, due to dysfunction of the sympathetic nervous system, the size of the patient's pupils can be grossly affected. Some patients have reduced sympathetic nerve activity leading to pupil constriction but having dilated pupils due to sympathetic overload is much more common, with the patient needing to avoid bright lights and sunshine. Some long COVID patients need to wear sunglasses all the time, with the worst cases so photophobic that they need to wear blackout eye masks.

The sooner that a long COVID patient receives a physical examination with confirmation of the definitive signs and symptoms of neurolymphatic dysfunction, the better. This hopefully will lead to a much quicker initiation of treatment than normal. The earlier the treatment programme begins, the better the chances of recovery and the less likely it is that the patient will start to spiral into the chronic severe state which is now affecting millions of long COVID patients worldwide, with the eventual diagnosis of ME/CFS and FMS.

At the time of writing this book, I have yet to see the same exact presentation in two patients. This is why this disorder is so confusing to most of the medical world as doctors can't place patients with long COVID into a box where they know exactly what diagnostic tests need to be done and what pills and potions need to be prescribed. Usually, all that the laboratory can achieve is to show that there are specific gene expressions or that some part of the patient's metabolism isn't working well and to exclude other diseases. The heterogeneity of the condition means that pharmacological treatment of long COVID is given for symptomatic relief but does not address the root biochemical cause, since every patient has their own unique biochemical pathway disruption.

By addressing the neuro-lymphatic pathway and improving the drainage of the central nervous system, one can achieve better long-term health in most sufferers of long COVID. As already explained, in disease states pain is often produced due to signals from sympathetic nerve fibres crossing over to adjacent sensory nerves in what are known as ephapses. This explains why in long COVID there seem to be quite random symptoms, not seemingly following a sensory nerve pathway. For instance, if you have a prolapsed intervertebral disc, commonly known as a 'slipped disc', in the lower lumbar spine at the base of your back, this would usually irritate and maybe even trap a nerve, or nerves, leading to pain radiating down the side and back of the thigh and down the lower leg to the feet.

This is due to an irritation of the sciatic nerve roots, leading to what many refer to as 'sciatica'. With long COVID, it is often the sympathetic nerves that are being irritated, in the thoracic spine and upper lumbar region. However, sensory nerves may also be irritated, spreading pain all over the back and down the extremities. This is why I sometimes see patients with 'crawling' sensations, numbness, tingling, pins-and-needles or stabbing pains in any part of their anatomy that cannot be simply explained when viewing the normal anatomical pathway of sensory nerves. One needs to examine the thoracic and upper lumbar regions of the spine, which is where the sympathetic nerves spread out from the spine to control the body, but much more importantly, receive messages from the body into the central nervous system.

This brings us to another long-held view in the medical world that has been turned virtually upside down by science. The autonomic nervous system for centuries has been looked on as mostly an efferent system – that is, one sending messages from the brain and the spine to the different parts of the body. For instance, sympathetic nerves generally control the circulation via efferent nerves sending messages to smooth muscle walls of the blood vessels. Very little importance has been placed on the afferent or sensory component of autonomic nerves, until the last few decades. In October 2016 Frank Willard, Professor of anatomy in Maine USA, lectured at the International Conference on Trauma, in Berlin, and discussed the work of neurophysiologist Professor Wilfrid Janig from Kiel University in Germany. Professor Janig believes that a major influence of sympathetic nerves is afferent, being much more important in the messages coming into the central nervous system.[15]

This is why the thoracic-spinal component of the Perrin Technique™ (see Chapter 4) is so important in both the examination and diagnosis. It is also why treatment to this region is a seminal part of the Perrin Technique™, especially the region where the sensory nerves enter the spinal cord, known as the dorsal root ganglia. The treatment of this region will be discussed in more detail in subsequent chapters. However, three tragic cases of ME/CFS patients in the UK offer physical proof that the dorsal root ganglia are affected in neuro-lymphatic disorders such as long COVID.

- **Lynn Gilderdale** was bedbound with ME for 17 years and took her own life in 2008. Whilst still a minor, Lynn was held in a secure unit at Guy's Hospital London until the medics requested permission to use force on her. Her parents refused and discharged her. This case was brought to the world stage by the terrible events following Lynn's assisted suicide, when her mother Kay was accused of her murder. Thankfully, Kay was acquitted and went on to write a moving book about this awful tragedy (*The Last Goodbye*). When Lynn's body was examined post mortem, inflammation of the dorsal root ganglia was discovered.

- **Sophia Mirza**: Similar findings were also discovered in 75% of the spinal cord during a post-mortem examination of this patient, organised by Criona Wilson, the courageous mother of Sophia Mirza, who tragically died in 2005 at the age of 32 from acute renal failure after suffering severely from ME/CFS for six years (see www.sophiaandme.org.uk). Sophia's death was the first ever case to have ME/CFS officially recorded as a contributing factor in the cause of death.

- **Merryn Crofts**: More recently, at an inquest in May 2018, 21-year-old Merryn Crofts, who had tragically died the year before, became the second person in the UK to have ME/CFS officially recorded as a causative factor in her death. Merryn's family donated her brain and spinal column for research and dorsal root ganglionitis was yet again discovered in her spine.

Fatigue in long COVID

Fatigue is a very common symptom in long COVID and is often regarded by practitioners as being psychogenic in origin, resulting from severe physical and/or mental activity, or lack of sleep. The degree of the fatigue will vary according to the personality and stamina of the individual.

To explain what is happening, experiments have shown, for example, that if a movement of the hand is continued for long enough to initiate a state of fatigue, and if at this stage the blood flow into the hand is stopped by inflating a cuff around the upper arm, although the somatic motor nerves are still functioning, there is no recovery of power until the cuff is released and normal circulation is restored.[16]

The blood flow to the muscles is under the influence of the sympathetic nervous system. Thus, if the sympathetic nerves are not functioning correctly, it could lead to a reduced blood flow to certain muscles. One would then reasonably assume that these muscles would be likely to suffer from some form of fatigue.

In long COVID, the normal activity within the sympathetic nervous system breaks down, as we have seen in Chapter 1. The effect may be systemic, causing widespread aches and pains throughout the entire body, or it may limit the fatigue to one or two muscle groups.

As we discussed in Chapter 1, the sympathetic nervous system also controls the lymphatic system and in long COVID the dysfunction of the sympathetic nervous system leads to a backflow of toxins.

As anybody taking part in sports, especially endurance athletes such as marathon runners or road cyclists, knows, when muscles have been over-working for too long, they may get cramps, possibly severe spasms and pain. This is due to a build-up of lactic acid. When we exert ourselves, we begin to breathe faster to supply more oxygen to the body. There are two forms of exercise: aerobic (using oxygen) and anaerobic. As long as we breathe and exercise gently, we use oxygen, which combined with glucose produces the energy needed by our working muscles. During exertion, the body may not deliver enough oxygen to supply the extra demand, which leads to anaerobic respiration.

This process yields energy from glucose being broken down into a substance called pyruvate which, in the absence of oxygen, converts into a substance called lactate. Lactate allows glucose breakdown and thus energy production to continue. The working muscle cells can continue this type of anaerobic energy production at high rates for only a couple of minutes, before high levels of lactate amass.

High lactate levels lead to an increase in the acidic state of the substance – that is, lactic acid. The high acidity within the muscle cells leads to disruptions of other metabolites. The same metabolic pathways that permit the breakdown of glucose to energy perform poorly in this acidic environment. This prevents permanent damage during extreme exertion by slowing the key systems needed to maintain muscle contraction. Once the body slows down, oxygen becomes available and lactate reverts back to pyruvate, allowing continued aerobic metabolism and energy for the body's recovery from the strenuous event.

Contrary to popular opinion, lactate or lactic acid build-up is not responsible for the muscle soreness felt in the days following strenuous exercise. Rather, the production of lactate and other metabolites during extreme exertion results in the burning sensation often felt in active muscles (a 'stitch'), though which exact metabolites are involved remains unclear. This often-painful sensation also gets us to stop overworking the body, thus forcing a recovery period in which the body clears the lactate and other metabolites.

An earlier clinical trial that I carried out with colleagues at the University of Central Lancashire concluded that a possible major cause of the muscle fatigue in ME/CFS is lack of lymphatic drainage of the muscle due to sympathetic dysfunction. This would lead to an excess of lactic acid among other metabolites in the muscles of ME/CFS patients.[17]

In 2013, researchers in Newcastle, UK, showed, using advanced brain scanning technology, that disturbance in cerebral vascular control associated with sympathetic dysfunction in the brain is directly related to excess lactic acid in skeletal muscle leading to fatigue in ME/CFS. The cells from ME/CFS patients produced on average 20 times as much lactic acid when exercised, suggesting an underlying cause for the aching muscles that patients often experience as soon as they begin to exercise. 'We have found very real abnormalities', said Professor Julia Newton, the head of the research.[18]

Muscles, like other tissues of the body, need a healthy lymphatic system, otherwise there will be no way of dealing with the excess lactic acid that Newton and her colleagues discovered. If the drainage was going in the wrong direction it would lead to further increase of lactic acid and metabolites in the muscles and further pain and discomfort. Elevated lactate levels have also been found in patients with fibromyalgia,[19] and in a new study at Vrije University in Amsterdam, Dutch scientists have shown that there is widespread damage in muscles of long COVID patients, with evidence of dysfunctional mitochondria, abnormal oxygen uptake in the muscles, blood clotting, altered immune response with an abnormal build-up of T-lymphocytes leading to further autoimmune-like muscle tissue damage, and an increase in lactic acid.[20]

A reversal of lymph drainage would explain the build-up of excess lactic acid, surplus levels of T-lymphocytes plus the increased clotting due to too an overabundance of fibroblasts in the blood.

In a new study led by Professor of Immunology, Onur Boyman, of the University of Zurich, which has just been published as I finish this book, the blood of long COVID patients was shown to have complement system dysregulation with excess complement proteins and more clotting factors.[21]

About 50 proteins make up the complement system and are a major part of the innate immune system. Activation of the complement triggers a cascade of reactions that produce different fragments which perform various functions that help fight infections and stimulate the inflammatory process.

The complement of protein molecules needs to be decommissioned and drained away from the site of infection otherwise it will lead to chronic inflammation and autoimmune response with the excess proteins causing healthy tissue to be harmed.

A healthy lymphatic system is required to drain the toxins out of harm's way and to stop the inflammatory reaction. If this process is not working correctly in the right direction, the result will be exactly what Onur Boyman and his team have found in patients, as he states: 'with long COVID, the complement system no longer returns to its basal state'. So, on top of the increase in clotting of the blood a patient has an immune reaction that is out of control.

One of the main roles of the lymphatic system is the transport of fat. With a reversal of normal drainage of lipids in long COVID, there will also be an increase of lipid mediators in the blood. Many mediators of inflammation are derived from phospholipids and polyunsaturated fatty acids, including prostaglandins, leukotrienes and platelet-activating factor, leading to the clots and thrombosis seen in long COVID.[22]

Exercise often helps fatigue associated with an overall lack of fitness resulting in deconditioning and also with depression, but excessive activity always exacerbates fatigue in patients with long COVID. In fact, too much physical activity can trigger a relapse in someone who is on the road to recovery. The simple question every practitioner needs to ask when initially examining a possible long COVID patient is, 'Does exertion ever improve the symptoms, or does it aggravate the condition?' If the latter is true, it is probably long COVID even if at the time of exertion, the patient feels good but then suffers afterwards.

Types of fatigue: post-exertional malaise (PEM) and post-exertional neuro-immune exhaustion (PENE)

Professor David Putrino, the director of rehabilitation innovation for Mount Sinai Health System based in New York, is fighting the idea that long COVID patients are just fatigued due to deconditioning and welcomes this new research that shows there are real physical and pathophysiological changes going on. His general guidance, like mine, is to avoid exercise if you have post-exertional malaise (PEM) and instead conserve your energy.

In Putrino's clinic, patients with PEM are taught very gentle exercises to improve cardiovascular fitness and rehabilitate the autonomic nervous system.

It is also important to realise that this build-up of lactic acid in the muscles of long COVID patients follows exertion, with the effects often delayed until the patient tries to utilise the muscles later on. A pivotal study on ME/CFS by scientists in California demonstrated PEM only by testing and then re-testing the muscle the following day.[23]

Patients with long COVID all suffer from PEM. This differs from normal fatigue which is proportional to the intensity and duration of activity, followed by a quick restoration of energy.

PEM is the worsening of symptoms after physical or mental activity that would not have caused a problem before illness, with symptoms typically worsening 12 to 48 hours after activity and lasting for days or even weeks.

The French word *malaise* means 'ill at ease' from mal- ('bad, badly') + aise ('ease'). In other words, it is a vague term for a general feeling of discomfort, illness or fatigue that has no clearly identifiable cause. This is exactly what patients with long COVID experience, with different levels of severity from being a little 'off colour' to completely bedridden.

Professor Lenny Jason and colleagues at De Paul University, Chicago, found that when questioning participants in a study on ME/CFS, there was much confusion as to what PEM meant and how it differs from the term post-exertional neuro-immune exhaustion (PENE) used in the international criteria.[24]

PENE is defined in the international consensus criteria for ME/CFS as a pathological low threshold of physical and mental fatigability, exhaustion, pain, and an abnormal exacerbation of neuro-immune symptoms in response to exertion.[25] In PENE there is more emphasis on immune-related problems than the other long COVID symptoms. This differs totally from the usual beneficial effects of exertion in some psychiatric disorders, such as clinical depression.

It is important clinically to note that if the patient feels occasionally improved following exertion, there could be an element of clinical depression. However, the patient may be suffering from both conditions at one time.

People often confuse the term 'exertion' with 'exercise'. In clinic, when I ask a patient if exertion helps or worsens their condition, sometimes the patient will say they feel better after a stroll, or a gentle cycle. There are plenty of patients with less severe symptoms who do benefit from keeping active without overloading their bodies. This is not exertion! Exertion is when a person feels that they have pushed their body more than they can cope with. With long COVID, this will inevitably lead to the overall symptom picture worsening and, as Lily Chu and colleagues found out during a Stanford University research study, some patients with ME/CFS don't feel the post-exertional malaise immediately but only later on and in some cases three days after exerting themselves.[26] The same delay in PEM seems to affect many long COVID patients.

A positive approach is important in fighting any disorder, but the horrible irony of long COVID, as with ME/CFS, is that it usually affects people who are determined, positive characters who would usually beat most illnesses with willpower alone. It is no secret that a strong willpower has been shown to help combat all types of disease, even some potentially fatal conditions, such as cancer. The power of the mind appears to be a vital tool in overcoming pathology, by improving the immune system through neuro-immune connections. However, the neurological pathway that is involved in this phenomenon is part of the sympathetic nervous system, the very system that breaks down in long COVID. Thus, the more the patient tries to beat the illness by pushing themselves, the worse the symptoms become.

Some psychologists believe that patients with long COVID 'perceive' greater fatigue during exercise as a result of the interaction of psychological distress, physical de-conditioning and/or sleep disturbance. They believe that the patient's fear of making their symptoms worse may lead to their reducing their activity and that the resultant physical de-conditioning can spiral into chronic disability, which leads to adverse psychological effects. Graded activity is the process of gently increasing activity to counterbalance physical de-conditioning. Patients are expected to follow the prescribed exercises, irrespective of any worsening in the symptoms and to fight against their 'perceived' fatigue.

In a statement, the National Institute for Health and Care Excellence (NICE) that produces the guidelines for doctors in the UK, has said that it was aware of concerns related to the impact of graded exercise therapy (GET) for managing post-viral fatigue in patients recovering from COVID-19, noting that 'it may not be appropriate for this group of patients'.[27]

As Professor David Putrino stated in an interview with *Shots Health News* on 9 January 2024: 'We need to step out of this erroneous mindset of no pain, no gain.'[28]

Fatigue as an early predictor of long COVID

As I said in the Introduction to this book, I drafted a letter on the day the worldwide pandemic was announced by the World Health Organization on 11 March 2020. This letter was subsequently published in the *Journal of Medical Hypotheses.*[29]

My research colleagues Lisa Riste, Andreas Walther, Adrian Heald, Annice Mukherjee and Mark Hann and I wanted to highlight the potential for a post-viral syndrome to manifest following COVID-19 infection as previously reported following the severe acute respiratory syndrome (SARS) epidemic that occurred in 2003 in Hong Kong and Canada, also a coronavirus.[30]

After the acute SARS episode some patients, many of whom were health-care workers, went on to develop a myalgic encephalomyelitis/chronic fatigue syndrome (ME/CFS)-like illness which nearly 20 months on prevented them returning to work.[31] We proposed that once an acute COVID-19 infection had been overcome, a subgroup of remitted patients were likely to experience long-term adverse effects resembling ME/CFS symptomatology such as persistent fatigue, diffuse myalgia, depressive symptoms and non-restorative sleep.

Post-mortem SARS research indicated the virus had crossed the blood–brain–barrier into the hypothalamus via the olfactory pathway.[31] The pathway of the virus seemed to follow the same route that I had claimed was dysfunctional in

ME/CFS, involving disturbance of lymphatic drainage from the microglia in the brain.[32] One of the main pathways of the lymphatic drainage of the brain is via the perivascular spaces along the olfactory nerves through the cribriform plate into the nasal mucosa.[33]

If the pathogenesis of coronavirus affects a similar pathway, we argued, it could explain the loss of smell (anosmia) observed in a proportion of COVID-19 patients. This disturbance we claimed leads to a build-up of pro-inflammatory agents, especially post-infectious cytokines such as interferon gamma, and interleukin 7,[34] which I had originally hypothesised would affect the neurological control of the 'glymphatic system' as observed in ME/CFS.[32] As detailed in Chapter 3, the build-up of cytokines in the central nervous system may lead to post-viral symptoms due to pro-inflammatory cytokines passing through the blood–brain–barrier in circumventricular organs, such as the hypothalamus, leading to autonomic dysfunction manifesting acutely as a high fever and in the longer term to dysregulation of the sleep/wake cycle, cognitive dysfunction and profound unremitting anergia, all characteristics of ME/CFS.

As happened after the SARS outbreak, a proportion of COVID-19-affected patients, we suggested, would go on to develop a severe post viral syndrome we termed 'post COVID-19 syndrome' – a long-term state of chronic fatigue characterised by post-exertional neuro-immune exhaustion.[35] This state is now known worldwide as long COVID and 'the proportion' of patients developing the long-haul symptoms numbers over 65 million worldwide.[36]

By the time the letter was ready for publication I had already seen a patient with possible post-COVID-19 syndrome.

My first long COVID patient

My first long COVID patient was a 42-year-old man, married with five children, who had been fit and healthy with no prior existing symptoms, with the exception of mild anxiety 10 years previously, and a month of fatigue following a viral infection four years previously. He had contracted the virus and had symptoms from 3 to 15 April 2020, during which time he had been virtually bed-bound for about two weeks. At the end of April, he contacted my osteopathic clinic and when examined scored 164/324 regarding the severity of symptoms on the validated rating scale Profile of Fatigue Related States (PFRS).[37] The PFRS scale lists 54 symptoms, each with a score of 0–6, where 0 = no symptom, 3 = moderate and 6 = extreme. Twenty-four of his symptoms initially scored high, i.e. 4, 5 and 6 on the scale.

I saw him in clinic on 5 May 2020, complaining of severe physical fatigue, insomnia, difficulty reading with brain fog, general myalgia, dry skin and increased anxiety. On physical examination he had a restricted and inflamed mid-thoracic spine (see page 29), engorged varicose lymphatics in the chest (page 31) with severe tenderness in the left breast lateral and superior to the left nipple (page 32). I also found marked tenderness in his coeliac plexus and a disturbed cranial rhythmic impulse (page 37). As explained earlier in this chapter, these signs are useful in the diagnosis of ME/CFS.[32]

Three treatments of the Perrin Technique™ (described in Chapter 4) were completed, once a week, and he followed a self-massage routine to aid lymphatic drainage along with doing gentle exercises to improve his thoracic spinal mobility. By the third treatment (27 May) the severity of his symptoms had reduced significantly, with a follow-up PFRS score of 75/324 with all but five of the very severe symptoms relating to physical and mental fatigue now being reduced from 4, 5 or 6 to only mild/moderate complaints, i.e. 1–3 on the severity scale.

Our conclusions

I and my colleagues concluded that it might be that early intervention and supportive treatments at the end of the acute phase of COVID-19 can help overcome acute phase symptoms and prevent them becoming longer-term consequences. Without this, we predicted in a contracted future economy (at least in the short to intermediate term), managing these likely post-COVID-19 syndrome cases, in addition to existing ME/CFS cases, would place additional burden on our already hard-pressed healthcare system.

In the light of this and similar cases and in the context of the available evidence for SARS, we suggested that priority should be given to examining the prevalence of fatigue-related symptoms following COVID-19 infection and to explore pragmatic relatively low-cost techniques to treat post-viral fatigue, to alleviate symptoms and improve the quality of life for those affected by the longer term sequelae of COVID-19. We concluded with a rally to the medical world in 2020: *'Let's start the preparations now for what may come in due course.'*

My Manchester University research group followed the above paper with a small study titled 'Reducing fatigue-related symptoms in long COVID-19: a preliminary report of a lymphatic drainage intervention'. This was published in the *Journal of Cardiovascular Endocrinology and Metabolism* in June 2022.[38]

In this study we presented an analysis of a case series of the first 20 patients' data collected in clinical practice to evaluate the potential of the Perrin Technique™ for long COVID.

Face-to-face treatment sessions with Perrin Technique™ practitioners occurred weekly involving effleurage/other manual articulatory techniques. The individuals being treated also undertook daily self-massage along with gentle mobility exercises following the advice in Chapter 7 of this book. Patients recorded symptom severity using the self-report 54-item profile of fatigue-related states (PFRS) before and after treatment. The mean age of male patients was 41.8 years (range, 29–53 years), and for female patients, 39.3 years (range, 28–50 years). None of the participants had a prior diagnosis of chronic fatigue syndrome, and all were new attendees to the clinics at the time of initial assessment. The average number of treatment sessions was 9.7 in men and 9.4 in women. The reduction in PFRS scores was 41.8% in men and 60.5% in women. The highest subscale scores on average were for fatigue, with the lowest for somatic symptoms. All subscale scores showed, on average, a similar reduction of approximately 50% post intervention, with the reduction in score relating to a decrease in the severity of symptoms.

Our findings suggested that the Perrin Technique™ may help to reduce fatigue symptoms related to long COVID, perhaps preventing acute symptoms through early intervention.[38]

The problem with the cases mentioned above and the patients we are seeing at present is that most of the long COVID patients coming for treatment now have been ill for at least a year, with some being diagnosed with long COVID over three years ago and having progressively worsened as the days have turned to weeks and weeks to months with all the many symptoms growing in number and severity in the unfortunate patient.

However, on the plus side, as time goes on there are many new findings from different research scientists around the world that are building up an evidence base that backs up everything we hypothesised in our original paper. This hopefully will lead to more practitioners understanding the science behind my techniques and eventually realising that the Perrin Technique™ has a role to play in the global fight against long COVID. Belgian psychiatrist and researcher Dr Peter Wostyn MD[39] suggested a hypothesis for a possible pathophysiological mechanism underlying post-COVID-19 fatigue syndrome, which indicated a more profound destruction of the olfactory epithelium, resulting in death of a larger number of olfactory receptor neurons. Such major loss of olfactory receptor neurons may lead to reduced CSF drainage to nasal mucosa via the cribriform plate.

Long COVID and comorbidities

Many other disorders can cause symptoms similar to long COVID. Most sufferers of long COVID reading this will hopefully have had extensive tests to eliminate the possibility of a wrong diagnosis. Long COVID should only be judged to be the cause of the patient's symptoms when these other diseases have been ruled out, and all other possible explanations have been explored. Although long COVID is always a possibility after being infected by the COVID-19 virus, one should always ensure that no other serious condition is at the root of the problems being experienced.

The effect on the body from neurological and hormonal changes following long-term wear and tear is known as allostatic load. How the body achieves balance via the endocrine and neuro-immune mechanisms and copes with these changes is known as allostasis. The control of the natural balance of metabolic pathways in the body, i.e. homeostasis, is orchestrated by the autonomic nervous system, with the hypothalamus at the helm. Therefore, any aspect of metabolism can be disturbed when the hypothalamic function is directly affected by what is referred to as allostatic load, which may take the form of any type of stress or disease process, and this is precisely what is going wrong in long COVID.

There are many tests that can be carried out to confirm or exclude the most common disturbances in the body that can lead to a state of fatigue, for example.

If these tests show that a patient has levels that are very high or very low compared to the norms, it usually means that something else is going wrong as well as long COVID. However, they can also reveal changes in one or more elements within the blood that may reflect long-term health problems that are directly due to long COVID. For instance, a blood test could show that the patient's thyroid T4 (the hormone thyroxine) levels are low. This could be due to a separate condition that the patient has, but in many cases of long COVID it reveals dysfunction of the hypothalamus, which leads to it sending the wrong messages to the pituitary gland, which in turn fails to regulate the amount of thyroxine that is produced by the thyroid gland in the neck, leading to a disturbance of many metabolic functions, such as heart rate, and can be a cause of fatigue.

Metabolic dysfunction can lead to many other conditions that occur together with long COVID, but the existence of comorbidities should not exclude a diagnosis of long COVID.

To be fair, diagnostic criteria are often developed for research purposes only and not really intended for clinical use. In research studies, it is imperative that you do not include comorbidities, otherwise you do not know if a treatment procedure tested is affecting the specific illness. However, in clinical situations, as I have explained, comorbidities should never lead to excluding the diagnosis of long COVID.

It is equally wrong to assume that all symptoms are a result of long COVID. A patient may have two, three or even more conditions affecting their body at the same time causing similar symptoms; this makes treatment more difficult and usually worsens the prognosis of the illness. The multiple illness case scenario in long COVID is much more common than people think and increasingly I am called upon to treat patients with what I call long COVID+.

So, what are the common comorbidities with long COVID? All the conditions discussed below that can also cause fatigue and other similar symptoms are found occasionally together with ME/CFS, which can, as I have said, be very confusing for the practitioner, since it isn't always clear which condition is responsible for the individual symptoms. The same can definitely be said for patients with long COVID.

As I put the finishing touches to my book it has just been announced that maverick US senator Bernie Sanders is leading the charge calling for a $10 billion research grant from the National Institute of Health into long COVID over the next 10 years. This new movement is known as the 'Long COVID Moonshot'.

The home page of their website[40] states:

'There are an estimated 18 million Americans suffering from Long Covid which is the equivalent of one in 18, and zero proven treatments. Many are too sick to leave their beds, work, or care for their family. Research funding is drying up and the U.S. has no additional plans to support clinical trials.

'The moonshot solution.

'Our campaign's primary goal is to achieve a minimum of $1B in annual funding for research and therapeutic clinical trials. Consistent research funding means a much better chance of getting us the treatment we need.'

However, many in the ME/CFS community have grave concerns that all the funding will go into long COVID and miss many other health problems.

Campaigner, health journalist and blogger Cort Johnson recently wrote in his award-winning *Health Rising* online resource:[41]

'There's enough room in this billion-dollar-a-year effort for other post-viral diseases. We don't need to leave anyone behind. The fix is so easy and this is the time to do that. Sanders has released a proposal – not a bill and there's still time to change it. We simply need to insert "and associated conditions" into the proposal.'

Together with the US patient advocate group, Solve ME, Johnson is trying to address this problem and change the proposal before it becomes a Bill.

The conditions Cort refers to are diseases such as POTS, ME/CFS fibromyalgia, post-treatment Lyme disease, mast cell activation syndrome (MCAS), and other complex, multi-systemic diseases which commonly cause very similar symptoms (see next). I believe they all share a fundamentally similar pathophysiology, affect millions of people and are very poorly funded by bodies such as the National Institutes of Health (NIH).

I, and many clinicians around the world, are starting to see in clinic patients with long COVID who additionally have the comorbidities discussed in the next section. Although these comorbidities have not yet been officially linked with long COVID, I most certainly feel there is often an overlap, so they should be carefully considered when diagnosing a patient.

Postural orthostatic tachycardia syndrome (POTS)

POTS occurs when the autonomic nervous system fails to compensate for upright body posture and causes fainting and dizziness due to low blood pressure on standing. The condition has been recognised since at least 1940, affecting millions worldwide aged 15–50 years, with a female to male ratio of around 5:1.[42, 43]

Professor Peter Rowe, a world-famous paediatrician, who is head of paediatrics at Johns Hopkins University Hospital in Baltimore, has found that many young patients with ME/CFS also have orthostatic intolerance and, in many cases, POTS.[44] The same presentations are being seen by Dr Rowe and his team in patients with long COVID.[45]

Researchers at the University of Newcastle, UK, studied haemodynamic responses of ME/CFS patients when standing for over two minutes. Professor Julia Newton, who led the research team, concluded that POTS was relatively common in ME/CFS patients, and patients' clinical evaluation should include autonomic function tests, such as the response to standing – POTS is indeed an under-recognised condition in ME/CFS.[46]

Diagnosis

POTS is confirmed by lying on a head-up tilt table (HUT) in a specialised clinic which is then tilted upright to a 60–80-degree vertical angle for approximately 45 minutes and blood pressure and heart rate are measured during this time.

The standing test is another test for POTS which can be done in any clinic, with the patient being asked to stand upright without any assistance, so s/he must support her/his own weight and maintain balance.

In long COVID, many patients suffer from orthostatic hypotension, also known as postural (standing up) hypotension (low blood pressure), which causes dizziness if one gets up too quickly from lying or sitting. This is due to disturbed sympathetic control leading to a blood pressure that is not high enough to pump sufficient blood into the head when standing up. This form of postural hypotension is also known as neurally-mediated hypotension. POTS is a more serious version of this problem and is diagnosed if the heart rate increases to 120 beats per minute or by 30 bpm (40 bpm in patients aged from 12 to 19) in 5 to 30 minutes after standing up, and the disorder has lasted at least six months with no other obvious cause of the symptoms, such as bleeding, other heart conditions or a side effect of medications.

Since the sympathetic nervous system mainly uses the neurotransmitter noradrenaline (norepinephrine) to transmit impulses, a high plasma level of noradrenaline seen in sympathetic disturbances is also considered useful to identify some POTS patients.[47]

Treatment

There is no universally accepted treatment for POTS, with some doctors prescribing beta blockers or steroids such as fludrocortisone, or some other medication to increase blood pressure, but there are many other non-pharmaceutical measures that may help.

People with POTS should eat small regular meals and drink 2 litres of fluids and increase salt intake to about 2–3 teaspoons a day.[48]

However, patients should avoid the increase in salt if they suffer from high blood pressure at other times or kidney problems. If in any doubt about health risks, it is best to check with their doctor before increasing their salt intake.

Orthostatic intolerance is common to many long COVID patients without full-blown POTS and is due to the effect on the autonomic control of blood pressure and volume caused by the shift of large amounts of blood volume from upper to lower body. It is traditionally treated with intravenous saline but this has complications if used in the long term.

Oral rehydration salts (ORS), which usually contain glucose plus sodium and potassium salts, are available online or from pharmacies as convenient sachets of pre-formulated low-concentration granules. These are effective, inexpensive, safe and convenient; when mixed with a litre of water they will rehydrate the body fast, regardless of the underlying problem. One should buy/recommend only those that follow the WHO formula – a tried-and-tested sodium and glucose mixture that has been used by the WHO in cholera outbreaks. Researchers in New York have shown that ORS improved short-term orthostatic tolerance exhibited by patients with POTS.[49]

However, some patients with long COVID have problems with their insulin levels or issues with excess yeast, such as candida, and risk aggravating the condition by the addition of glucose in any form, so patients should tread very carefully and again seek advice from their GP.

In long COVID, total inactivity will make the condition worse so it is important to try to maintain some muscle strength, especially in the legs. Consequently, regular gentle exercise even if it is just clenching the buttocks for a few minutes a day, will be of use. When the patient is lying down, the head end of their bed should always be raised and they should never get up quickly, which is also a golden rule for ME/CFS patients. Sit on the side of the bed for at least a minute before standing and always avoid long periods of standing still. Dizziness or feeling faint can be helped by lying down and raising the legs. If the patient is unable to lie down, they can cross their legs in front of each other while standing and squeeze their legs together, or rock up and down on their toes. Clenching other parts of the body, such as buttocks and tummy muscles and/or even the fists, may help, and in some cases compression tights may also help.

Joint hypermobility and Ehlers-Danlos syndrome (EDS)

Many patients seen in clinic with long COVID have extraordinary mobility in their joints. There are more and more cases of connective tissue disorders as a comorbidity of long COVID.[50]

The hypermobility is sometimes found to be due to EDS, which is now known to be a group of connective tissue disorders that are mostly inherited and are varied both in how they affect the body and in their genetic causes. EDS patients also may have skin that can be stretched much more than normal.

At the time of writing, EDS is classified into 13 subtypes. Each subtype is classified by slightly different clinical symptoms and identifiable variants in genetic testing. However, some patients are diagnosed as having EDS on signs and symptoms alone without a confirmed genetic abnormality.

Patients with EDS have loose/unstable joints which are prone to frequent dislocations and joint pain, hyper-extensible joints and often an early onset of osteoarthritis. The fragile skin may lead to severe bruising and scarring, with slow and poor wound healing. They may also have fragile arteries, intestines and uterus, and often have a poor spinal posture, with a thoracic spine which is bent forward with some side-bending (kyphoscoliosis), poor muscle tone, heart valve problems and gum disease.

Connective tissue is what the body uses to provide strength and elasticity and is found all over the body. Normal connective tissue contains strong proteins that allow tissue to be stretched but not beyond a certain limit, and then safely returns that tissue to normal. The connective tissue in EDS is badly constructed or processed, with some or all of the body affected, and can be pulled beyond normal limits, which causes damage to the tissue. Being a genetic disorder, the same symptoms run in families. (NB: There are some rare cases where the EDS has been a caused by genetic mutation and is not familial.)

There is an assessment tool used by many practitioners to confirm a hypermobility state. It is known as the Beighton scale[51] which is included below and gives scores related to the severity and extent of the hypermobility. However, the scale was developed as a research tool to indicate general hypermobility. Often a score over 6 is used as a diagnosis of generalised hypermobility but does not mean a person has EDS or any other disease process. Joints not evaluated on the Beighton scale can be hypermobile so sometimes a low score does not indicate the severity of the condition.

The Beighton score is calculated as follows:

- One point if, while standing, when bending forward you can place the palms of your hands on the ground with legs straight and no bending of the knees.
- One point for each elbow that bends backwards (extends) 10 degrees or more.
- One point for each knee that bends backwards (extends) 10 degrees or more.
- One point for each thumb that touches the forearm when bent backwards.
- One point for each little finger that bends backwards beyond 90 degrees.

The primary feature of EDS is abnormal connective tissue, which can also affect the walls of blood vessels, leading to veins distending excessively in response to ordinary pressures from the blood flow. This in turn leads to increased pooling of blood in swollen veins and many associated symptoms. These include frequently fainting or feeling very dizzy all the time, especially when standing still and even worse in a hot shower. Connective tissue disorders can also affect the integrity of lymphatic vessels and may also contribute to the backflow of lymph and varicose megalymphatics (grossly enlarged lymph vessels – see page 31) and sometimes stretch marks seen in long COVID patients.

Cranio-cervical instability (CCI)

In some severe cases of EDS there is also the possibility of cranio-cervical instability (CCI), also known as occipito–atlanto–axial (OAA) hypermobility syndrome or atlanto–axial instability (AAI). This condition is the due to weakness and hyperlaxity of ligaments that join the occipital bone at the bottom of the skull with bones at top of the neck. The first cervical vertebra is also known as the atlas and the second, the axis. Instability in this region may lead to damage and dysfunction of the upper part of the spinal cord or, worse, the brain itself. One of the structural effects seen in AAI can be a Chiari malformation, which is where there is a downward displacement of part of the cerebellum at the base of the brain. The diagnosis of CCI/AAI is usually made following an upright MRI and rotational three-dimensional CT scans and then confirmed by a reduction of symptoms when the head is gently pulled up from the neck and worsened by pushing the head gently down. Other physicians and neurosurgeons, such as Dr Dan Heffez of Wisconsin, USA, have seen the connection between FMS and Chiari malformation and upper cervical problems,[52] but besides anecdotal evidence at this time (April 2024) this link hasn't been reported on in any scientific paper about long COVID.

For most cases of early stage CCI, I recommend a soft cervical collar to be used for an hour at a time on the front part of which the patient can rest their chin comfortably, taking the strain off the upper neck. This should be used in combination with frequent applications of cold and warm compresses ('contrast bathing'), as mentioned in Chapter 4 (page 100). Very gentle specific isometric exercises are also given in Chapter 7, which will gradually strengthen the suboccipital region. The exercises need to be done in very short, gentle bursts but have to be carried out frequently, at around every three hours throughout the day, and as with all exercises for long COVID, they must be painless. If even the slightest tightening of the muscles elicits pain, then the patient should stop. As I say to all my students in my workshops: 'PAIN = NO GAIN'. Pain is the enemy of long COVID as the neural pain pathways will aggravate already aggravated pain control centres in the brain.

There are practitioners who have successfully treated more severe CCI for years without surgery. They use a type of injection technique for joint hypermobility known as prolotherapy. It utilises a sclerosing injection which is designed to irritate the joint and sounds like it shouldn't help because, as it says on the bottle, it irritates the joint! How can this oxymoron be explained? With a skilled practitioner the injection, which usually has an analgesic and possibly an anti-inflammatory component, will also contain a saline or sucrose solution which, by irritating the ligaments, causes them to tighten, resulting in an improvement in joint strength and less hypermobility.

Some practitioners use prolozone injections, which contain ozone to achieve the same results as prolotherapy, but which practitioners claim is a quicker method with fewer side effects.

Idiopathic intracranial hypertension (IIH)

IIH, previously known as 'benign intracranial hypertension' or 'pseudotumor cerebri', is a condition of unknown cause leading to an increase in pressure within the brain.

Like long COVID , it most commonly affects women and leads to daily diffuse, non-pulsating head pain which is aggravated by coughing. The most common finding is papilloedema, which is an eye condition that happens when pressure in the brain makes the optic nerve swell, affecting vision. However, recent research has looked into the possibility of a lesser, more common form of IIH, causing headaches and other symptoms but not papilloedema. A group of doctors who carried out research at Cambridge University have highlighted that this could explain many of the symptoms of ME/CFS and thereby of long COVID.[53]

The rationale behind this idea makes so much sense. Higgins and colleagues have argued that the most common presentation of most known diseases is always the mild form of the disorder. Asthma, for instance, it is a very common condition and affects many people who need the occasional puff on an inhaler but can manage their life without too many problems. However, there are some very severe manifestations that can hospitalise patients and even be a cause of death; thankfully these are much fewer than the minor cases. However, with the present accepted criteria for IIH, the more severe cases when there is headache and papilloedema and severe nausea, are the cases usually diagnosed, with less severe cases without papilloedema rarely diagnosed. This is very unlikely to be the true representation of the condition, and therefore there must be many people with minor forms of IIH never correctly diagnosed.

The Cambridge team had already shown in 2013 that some ME/CFS patients had symptom relief following a drainage of cerebrospinal fluid (CSF) using a lumbar puncture.[54] Although the lumbar puncture demonstrated the elevated intracranial pressure in the ME/CFS patients, in most cases I would not recommend sticking a needle into the spinal cord to remove fluid as it could worsen the condition due to the risk of damaging the subarachnoidal lymphatic-like membrane (SLYM) that has recently been discovered (see Chapter 6, page 150). Lumbar punctures have actually caused a major relapse in the symptoms of many of my ME/CFS patients over the years who have had this procedure for investigative purposes only. However, in some severe cases of long COVID when nothing else is working and the patient presents with unremitting headache with nausea, a lumbar puncture may be worth considering as a final option with the doctor performing the procedure being very careful not to push the needle through the SLYM.

IIH has been clearly demonstrated in some patients with ME/CFS and has also been identified in FMS by a group of Belgian researchers.[55] Thakur and colleagues have already detected a link between COVID-19 and some patients with IIH.[56]

This view that at least a subgroup of COVID-19 patients may represent a variant of IIH is supported by a very recent study by Silva and colleagues who described the characteristics of headache and the CSF profile during SARS-CoV-2 infection in a consecutive series of COVID-19 patients. The authors excluded those who presented any clinical or laboratory evidence for meningitis or meningoencephalitis and concluded that the headache was due to intracranial hypertension in the absence of meningitic or encephalitic features,[57] so it is only a matter of time before we see more long COVID patients with IIH as a possible comorbidity.

Fibroblasts and long COVID

One of the main problems affecting many patients with long COVID is the fibrotic tissue formation in lungs, heart and many other organs. Fibroblasts are cells that are involved in the building, and maintenance and defence of organ tissue; they are involved in the synthesis of extracellular matrix, the network of macro-molecules, such as collagen and minerals that provide structure and biochemical support for adjoining cells. During normal repair processes, the fibroblasts are used up as the tissue repair resolves to form a scar. In pathological fibrosis the fibroblasts overproduce the extracellular matrix disturbing normal function of the organ and can lead to organ failure.

Because the control of lymph drainage is dysfunctional and reversed in long COVID, the protein molecules in the matrix accumulate in the tissues, leading to further fibrosis (hardening) and a greater danger of further infection. Also lining all vessels along the endothelium is part of the cellular matrix that forms a protective barrier of tissue known as the glycocalyx. The toxins building up could damage this important part of the integumentary system, which is the body's first line of defence, a physical barrier preventing entry of foreign material into the cell. The endothelial glycocalyx is a network of membrane-bound proteoglycans and glycoproteins, large protein molecules that cover the endothelium lumin. Both endothelium- and plasma-derived soluble molecules integrate into this mesh. If damaged, the glycocalyx requires a healthy lymphatic system to drain the macro-molecular proteins away from the tissue, otherwise there will be a build-up of the cellular matrix as mentioned above.[58]

Several viruses have been reported to infect fibroblasts. As stated below, ACE2 is a binding receptor of COVID-19. In COVID-19, the infection may cause a proliferation of fibroblasts and extracellular matrix over-production in the lungs.

Fibroblasts, as well as producing pro-inflammatory cytokines and causing T-cell infiltration, can enter the blood from the surrounding tissue via the damaged endothelium, including the glycocalyx, forming blood clots. ACE-2 fibroblasts may invade immune cells making them more prone to further viral infections.[59]

In addition to stimulating the lymph flow to drain the correct way and help rid the body of excess fibroblasts via the Perrin Technique™ these patients need a balanced modulated immune system which can be helped by two major plant-based wonders, flavanols and phytosterols. These compounds can be found in supplements containing turmeric, ginger, garlic, liquorice root and astragalus, and are discussed in detail in Chapter 9.

Obviously, any medication, even over-the-counter supplements and antihistamines, should only be taken after individual advice from your healthcare provider and/or pharmacist.

Conclusion

This chapter has shown that long COVID is caused by a predisposing dysfunction of the healthy flow of the neuro-lymphatic system, often due to spinal mechanics and cranial structure being disturbed, most likely many years before COVID-19 evolved. This in turn leads to the toxic overload of the central nervous system triggered by the SARS-CoV-2 virus; the vicious circle that ensues eventually leads to the chronic condition, which can be complicated by other related conditions.

Chapter 3

The role of toxins
in long COVID

'If you drink much from a bottle marked "poison" it is certain to disagree with you sooner or later.'

Lewis Carroll

Alice's Adventures in Wonderland, p. 11

Case: Karin's story

Infection with COVID: December 2022. After the symptoms like sore throat, severe cough, and strong headaches had improved a few weeks after the illness, new symptoms appeared that would then accompany me for many months: constant ear pain on the left side, nausea, shortness of breath due to limited lung function, sleep disorders, cognitive impairment (brain fog), palpitations, extreme tension in the neck and back, and total exhaustion even with handling everyday tasks at home. Crash situations – for example, when I had a doctor's visit – forced me to lie down for a whole week initially. In search of help, I visited numerous specialists, including alternative medicine practitioners, had various examinations (MRI), but no one could really help me, which almost made me despair. My family doctor then recommended a long COVID rehab, which I took advantage of in April 2023. Finally, I was cared for by doctors and therapists who took me and my conditions seriously and wanted to help me further. A patient, who was also affected, told me about the Perrin Technique™, which had helped her a lot. That's how I found Mr Nikolaus Altmann, and his clear diagnosis and prognosis gave me new hope!

For over six months, I went for treatment every week, then every second week, and now, after a year, every third week. With the support of my partner, who drove me to the treatment sessions, it was possible for me to get to Krems, Austria. Soon, I could notice improvements: first, my concentration improved, and the brain fog gradually cleared up. The ear pain and tension also became lighter. My resilience increased step by step, and I got better control over the exhaustion. Crash situations lasted only a few days, and after a few weeks, even less. The psychological component was also very important to me: through the weekly reflection and discussion of the current situation with Mr. Altmann, I had a good overview of my development and could track the progress well. Setbacks, which occurred repeatedly, were thus easier for me to handle. The Perrin treatments kept me optimistic, and I always believed that I would recover.

I understood that self-treatment was important for recovery, but I must honestly admit that it was difficult to carry it out regularly. At least, I occasionally did the facial and head massage, which was easier to incorporate into daily life.

The biggest stress factors during this time were not being taken seriously with long COVID symptoms or being pushed into the psychological corner. Moreover, it was a great burden that I was on sick leave for over a year and couldn't tell my employer when I would be fit for work again. Ultimately, I was prematurely retired.

This pressure was enormous, but here too, the Perrin treatments were always helpful. I was, and am, lucky to receive a lot of support from my partner and a few close friends. In the meantime, I can go for walks again, have started singing in the choir again, which is very good for me (also for my lung function), enjoy working in the garden, and meet friends again. However, always with an eye on what is possible and without overdoing it regarding the duration and intensity of my activities.

Karin R, Austria (translated from German)
Patient of osteopath and licensed Perrin Technique™
practitioner Nik Altmann, Austria

The word 'toxin' was coined in the late nineteenth century and is defined as 'an antigenic poison or venom of plant or animal origin, especially one produced or derived from micro-organisms, and causing disease when present at low concentrations in the body'.[1] For simplicity, 'toxin' is used in this book in the broader sense of any substance that is harmful to the body. For instance, mercury, which is a heavy metal, is from neither plant nor animal source but is nevertheless a major toxin to the body. Nowadays there are many man-made toxins, including artificial sweeteners such as aspartame and perfluorinated compounds (PFCs) such as Teflon.

The human body is designed to clear toxins that arise from its own metabolism and that come from the external sources, such as those I will describe below in detail. The liver, gastrointestinal system and the urinary system are essential in this process, but so too is the lymphatic system as I explain in greater detail in Chapter 4 (see Fact 2: Getting the toxins out, page 92). When the body's ability to get rid of toxins is compromised or the level of exposure is too great to be coped with, then symptoms of overload arise.

Toxins from within and without

To stay healthy we need to deal with toxins from two distinct sources: from inside and from outside the body.

Alongside the onslaught of thousands of manmade and natural chemical pollutants (see below) that harm the environment and do major damage to our bodies when we breathe in, drink or eat anything, our body may produce its own array of microbes and chemicals that can be toxic to ourselves. An example of this is the over-production of pro-inflammatory chemicals, such as cytokines, which are required to aid the body's immune system. If these, or any of the neurochemicals naturally produced in the central nervous system, are overactive, it can lead to neurotoxic effects. These can vary depending on which area of the spinal cord or brain are influenced by the excess chemicals produced.

An array of different chemicals that are produced in the body occur in a condition that is becoming increasingly seen in long COVID patients – namely, mast cell activation syndrome (MCAS). A mast cell is a type of white blood cell with many granules containing the chemical mediators histamine and tryptase, the most common enzyme found in mast cell prostaglandins. Histamine is a nitrogen-containing chemical that has properties influencing the body in many different ways, including affecting smooth muscle in the body – for instance, in the walls of blood and lymphatic vessels. When mast cells are activated by an allergen, they also release our old friends the pro-inflammatory cytokines such as TNF-alpha and certain prostaglandins, with prostaglandin D2 (PGD2) being the predominant prostaglandin product released by mast cells. If too many cytokines and prostaglandins are released they become toxic to the body.

Although best known for their role in allergies, mast cells are important in protecting the body by supporting the immune response. They are the only blood cells found throughout the brain, communicating with neurons and glial cells, and they also help the blood–brain barrier (BBB) function correctly.

The National Institute of Health in the USA has discovered a genetic abnormality that leads to high levels of tryptase. It is during MCAS that these and other mediators are over-produced, creating an over-active allergic response. This leads to an array of symptoms such as rashes like urticaria, more commonly known as hives, swelling, flushing, itching, abdominal pain, nausea/vomiting, loose bowels and difficulty breathing, which are all strangely familiar to many long COVID patients.

As discussed in more detail in Chapter 9, Dr Paul Glynne has discovered the close connection between long COVID and MCAS and treats the condition accordingly.[2]

A diagnosis of MCAS is aided by blood or urine tests which show a higher level of mediators during symptomatic episodes. Treatment for MCAS is usually just to relieve the symptoms. Sometimes antihistamines and other drugs to reduce the release of the mediators from the mast cells are prescribed. In very severe cases, the patient may go into anaphylactic shock, which requires an immediate injection of adrenaline.

In recent years, researchers have found that prostaglandins cross into the brain and bind to a specific kind of receptor, called EP3, to cause fever. Research has shown that EP3 receptors are found in a tiny region in the hypothalamus, the size of a pin head, known as the 'median preoptic nucleus', that is crucial in causing fever.[3]

The median preoptic nucleus is found behind the eyes, where the optic nerves cross paths as they enter the brain. If the toxic drainage along the perivascular space in the optic nerve pathway is affected, then it could lead to a build-up of pro-inflammatory cytokines and prostaglandins around this nucleus, and in these patients will lead to feverish symptoms in long COVID. In other patients, where different regions of neuro-lymphatic drainage are affected, or if there are different neurotoxins involved, such as heavy metals, then the symptoms will be different, without noticeable symptoms of fever.

In fact, I have just made a remarkable discovery showing that most of my patients have an increase in deposits of metals in their nervous system and exhibit a phenomenon that will blow your mind.

Heavy metals have been used over the years in vaccines. Mercury poisoning had been implicated in problems with vaccinations in general. Mercury is present in the preservative thimerosal (also known as thiomersal) that used to be the most common preservative in stockpiled vaccines, such as for cholera, tetanus, typhoid and influenza. Thankfully most pharmaceutical companies have taken thimerosal out of vaccines, but for many the damage has already been done. In many people any leakage into the surrounding fascia during a vaccination injection could leave a permanent deposit of mercury in the tissue in the upper arm. I have found that if you take a very strong, small magnetic disc made of neodymium, available to buy online, and place it on the upper arm/shoulder it will stick to the skin at the point containing remnants of the mercury (see page 85*).

What is so surprising, is that the magnetic discs are strongly attracted to and stick on skin overlying the upper and mid thoracic spine of many of my ME/CFS and long COVID patients (see Plate 3(a)) and some even have a strong magnetic attraction in their forehead (see Plate 3(b)) above the region of the main brain drainage in the olfactory pathways through the cribriform plate. This supports my original theory that toxins, including heavy metals, build up around the spinal cord as well as the brain in ME/CFS. This is clear evidence of metals being deposited in these spinal and cranial regions and not draining away, leading to a build-up of metallic neurotoxicity in and around the spinal cord and the brain. This amazing observation needs to be further explored and I hope to research this magnetic spine and forehead phenomenon in a future study.

WARNING: Do not use these very strong magnets near any person who has had a pacemaker, nerve stimulators or any metal implants inserted into their body. Consult your doctor if you have any doubts.

Inflammation and the gastrointestinal system

Inflammation of the gut is common among long COVID patients and many have been diagnosed with irritable bowel syndrome. Allergic reactions to food containing gluten are common. The best known condition involving such a reaction is coeliac disease in which the structure of the small bowel is destroyed, with a flattening of the deeply folded villi of the gut wall, and diminished capacity to properly absorb many key nutrients from food. Generally, long COVID patients do not test positive for coeliac disease, but as explained above, many become sensitive to a variety of chemicals and foodstuffs, especially gluten.

When digestion is impaired, the larger peptide fragments that make up proteins in food are not broken down. Among these are opioid peptides derived from two principal sources: casein in milk (the casomorphins) and gliadin in gluten (the gliadomorphins), which occur in wheat and other cereal crops, such as rye and barley. Opioids are peptides that have been found to possess morphine-like activity and are known to be naturally occurring in important transmitter molecules, particularly in the gut, brain and immune system.

When the gut wall has increased permeability, these opioid peptides, which would normally be kept inside the gut, are absorbed and act both locally in the gut and in other organs, particularly the brain. The same factors that render the gut permeable appear to increase the permeability of the blood–brain barrier (BBB) and allow access of these compounds to the brain.

Depending on the concentration of opioids in the gut, as well as the permeability of the gut wall and BBB, the overall level of these compounds in the bloodstream and the brain may be unstable and give rise to variable expressions of symptoms and dysfunction. Opioids play a significant part in the immune response through receptors found on cells of the immune system. Generally, they suppress the immune response and increase susceptibility to infection. The gut and the brain communicate via messenger molecules generated by the immune response.

The gut and brain also communicate neurologically. The enteric nervous system (ENS), which is an elaborate system controlling the whole gut, is connected to the central nervous system (CNS) through innervation by the autonomic nervous system, often referred to as the gut–brain axis. The ENS has been referred to as 'the second brain'. The gut has an intricate immune system network controlled by the ENS that produces a number of neurotransmitters, such as serotonin, acetylcholine and substance P. These have been shown to play a part in the communication between the gut and the brain and vice versa, and influence the activity of the gastrointestinal microbiota. It is now known that the gut's communication to the brain is as important as the messages from the brain to the gut.[4]

Messages between the brain and the rest of the body are modified by a regulatory action of the gut microbiota on the BBB converting from hormones into neurotransmitters in the brain, affecting control of the entire nervous system.

Lymphocytes involved in the immune response in the gut lead to the secretion of small amounts of hormones that are thought to play a local part in regulating inflammation in the gut. Due to the processes mentioned above, it is also possible that the release of hormones in the gut is influenced by stress and that problems affecting the gut and the brain may be a result of disrupted communications in the neuroimmune network.

It is now known that the microbiome helps produce around 70% of the neurotransmitters used in the brain. Unbelievably, over 90% of serotonin is produced in the gut. Serotonin is essential for feelings of wellbeing and is often the neurochemical targeted by antidepressants. Disruption of the gut microbiome can lead to an imbalance of serotonin and melatonin; melatonin is an essential component of the circadian rhythm, the 24-hour biological rhythm that regulates our sleep and wake cycles, in addition to many other important physiological processes.

In addition to the pineal gland in the brain, the gut is known also to produce melatonin. The microbiome has its own separate rhythm but is connected with the circadian rhythm; these two need to be in sync with each other, otherwise the person may be hungry and want to eat at all the wrong times for their body clock.

The role of the microbiome in neuroimmunology can explain why probiotics are so important following a short course of antibiotics, and imperative if one is prescribed long-term antibiotics for chronic bacterial illnesses such as Lyme disease. Many patients with long COVID have a history of repeated infections in their younger life, such as tonsilitis, requiring large amounts of antibiotics which would also reduce the quantity of good bacteria in the gut over time.

The gut-brain axis can equally be disturbed due to an excess of bacteria in the gut seen in the condition known as small intestinal bacterial overgrowth (SIBO), which also causes chronic diarrhoea, weight loss and malabsorption and is becoming more commonly identified.

Therefore as discussed above, with a dysfunctional lymphatic system which is pumping toxins in the wrong direction, neurochemicals and other large protein molecules, including hormones plus microbiota if overproduced, would not drain away and could have a toxic effect leading to many of the long COVID symptoms.

Pollutants

Environmental pollutants have long been seen as major causative factors in neurodegenerative disorders, such as Parkinson's disease, although there may also be genetic factors that make a person more susceptible to that illness. Studies have revealed major variations in an individual's ability to detoxify noxious agents and have shown that neurological disease may derive from an exceptional vulnerability to certain neurotoxins.

Amazingly, with over 144,000 chemicals in the environment, fewer than two dozen have actually been banned. The US Government Office of Technology has estimated that up to 25% of all chemicals might be neurotoxic.[7] The US Department of Health has estimated that each year approximately 2000 new chemicals are produced and, no matter what safety procedures are taken, they are all – inadvertently or deliberately – introduced into the environment via the air, water or foodstuffs.[8]

According to Julian Cribb, author of *Surviving the 21st Century*, more than 250 billion tonnes of chemical substances a year are harming people and life everywhere on the planet.[9] Worse still, Cribb notes that according to the World Health Organization, around 12 million people die every year from diseases caused by the direct and indirect impact of man-made pollutants. The figures per year are frightening.[9]

- 30 million tonnes of manufactured chemicals are produced per year.
- 400 million tonnes of hazardous waste are generated per year.
- Over 11 billion tonnes of coal, oil and gas are burned per year.

Not to mention the hundreds of billions of tonnes of waste products that are found in water and the food chain worldwide. Cribb comments that environmental pollutants have been discovered at the top of Mount Everest and at the bottom of the deepest oceans. Mercury is seen in the tissue of polar bears in the Arctic, and honeybees are dying globally from agricultural pesticides.[9]

I am not suggesting, as some conspiracy theorists do, that COVID-19 is a hoax, and that it is toxic exposure that is the cause of the deaths around the world. However, just as the sources of toxic exposure, such as benzene from motor fuels, organophosphates in pesticides, chlorofluorocarbons (CFCs) in cleaning products and carbon monoxide, have been implicated as potential causative factors of ME/CFS, I do believe that long-term exposure to environmental pollutants leads to a build-up of toxicity within the central nervous system, and especially when the person's central lymphatic drainage is already compromised, with the final trigger being an infection with the COVID-19 virus leading to long COVID.

One case that comes to mind is a couple who were both suffering from severe symptoms of ME/CFS. They were not blood related and yet both had been ill for a few years. They had been living in the same house for 20 years with their own little herb and vegetable garden, with no factories, farms or large roads nearby and their own market garden was 100% organic. They were not living under a flight path and they both had jobs that did not involve any contact with toxins.

It seemed a very unusual case. However, toxic screening at a local lab of the aforementioned couple showed they both had high levels of nickel and cadmium in their blood samples. On questioning, I found out that when they moved into their home it was a new build and further investigation revealed that it was built on a landfill site. I enquired about what the estate was built on and it turned out that it was not so surprising they were being poisoned, as the house was directly on top of a demolished car battery factory! Nickel and cadmium are used in the production of rechargeable batteries and obviously there was a seepage from the factory ruins into the soil. Sadly, this husband and wife both had different previous mechanical problems that had compromised their neuro-lymphatic pathways. However, the large quantity of vegetables and herbs grown in this poisoned soil, and eaten for many years by this unfortunate couple, lay behind their illness.

It is therefore always worth considering whether there is an environmental predisposing factor to consider in any cases of long COVID in individuals within a household who are not blood relatives.

Effects of neurotoxins

Toxic chemical exposure can cause many serious conditions, including cardiovascular, kidney and endocrine diseases. The most common organ to be affected by toxins, however, is the brain, leading to fatigue, exhaustion, cognitive impairment, loss of memory, insomnia, depression, psychosis and other disturbing symptoms.[10]

There are several specialised regions in the brain that do not have a complete blood–brain barrier (BBB) and which interact closely with the cerebrospinal fluid. These seven zones, known as the circumventricular organs, are chemical-sensitive regions that may react with toxins, sending messages to other parts of the brain, especially the hypothalamus.

The hypothalamus controls the hormonal (endocrine) system via a mechanism called biofeedback. Basically, the hypothalamus 'tastes' the blood to check how much of any hormone needs to be released into the circulation. It then sends messages to endocrine organs around the body to increase or decrease levels of the many different hormones. Since hormones are made up of large protein molecules, the BBB, which normally protects against large toxic molecules, is extremely permeable in the region of the hypothalamus, which contains two separate circumventricular zones, the median eminence and the organ vasculosum. This allows the passage of specific protein-transport molecules that enable huge molecules to pass through the BBB. Thus, the most permeable region of the BBB is at the hypothalamus, facilitating its ability to monitor hormone levels in the blood.

Autonomic dysfunction has long been associated with many toxic substances, especially following exposure to organic solvents, with some people exhibiting signs and symptoms of peripheral neuropathy (nerve damage in the limbs, hands and feet).

Under normal conditions, most of the BBB protects the central nervous system from rapid fluctuations in levels of ions, neurotransmitters, bacterial toxins, growth factors and other substances. However, its permeability has been shown to be increased by stress.[11]

Each organ or tissue may act as a discrete target for some toxic substances, which may lead to dysfunction of the whole organism. Specific molecules within a particular cell type act as primary targets. Some neurons are less susceptible than others to toxic damage, leading to regions of the brain that are not as sensitive to toxins.

Diet and toxicity

Exposure to chemicals affects people in different ways depending on several factors. Diet plays a crucial part in the body's ability to withstand toxicity. Toxins can be produced from non-toxic foods that we eat, building up in the central nervous system, liver or kidneys.

Trace elements, which are often used as supplements for good health, may become toxic if ingested in too high a dose. One thinks of selenium, for example, as a promoter of health, but it may be taken up from the soil by certain plants, such as species of the *Astralagus* genus, in sufficient quantities to render those plants toxic. Chronic selenium poisoning in animals, known as alkali disease, leads to cases of livestock with lameness, lack of vitality, hair loss, depressed appetite and emaciation.[12]

Healthy food may not be properly digested or absorbed. The person may have a leaky gut due to problems with the intestinal wall, leading to semi-digested food entering the bloodstream, causing immune responses which create further toxicity.[13, 14] Even fruit and vegetables, especially non-organic ones bought in supermarkets, often contain a cocktail of toxic chemical preservatives and enhancements which will aggravate the situation.

Damage to the lining of the alimentary canal (gut) may be caused by a variety of irritants, the most common being alcohol, aspirin, gluten and the yeast *Candida albicans*.[15] Deficiencies in some vitamins, proteins, essential fatty acids and minerals are known to lead to poor intestinal cell growth, causing increased permeability of the gut wall.[16] The gut's microbiome (resident bacteria and other microbes) is essential for the production of most of the chemicals used by the nervous system.

Toxins in the gut can destroy many of the 'good' bacteria and render the body incapable of producing the essential neuropeptides necessary for a healthy brain. This further exacerbates the toxic soup building up in the central nervous system in patients with a compromised neuro-lymphatic drainage. Add one final trigger to the equation, namely COVID-19, and the build-up of inflammatory chemicals such as cytokines following the acute infection will lead to the condition known as long COVID.

Neuro-inflammation

Whilst inflammation may not always affect the spine in long COVID and, in some cases, can only be found in some parts of the brain, there is now much evidence to support my original theory that pro-inflammatory cytokines and other neurotoxins pass through the BBB and into the glial cells of the brain, leading to neuro-inflammation.[14]

Neuro-inflammation is a symptom of many diseases, including Alzheimer's disease, Parkinson's disease and multiple sclerosis.[17] It has also been shown to be caused by disturbance in the neurotransmitters produced by the brain.[18] Other scientists have made similar claims regarding ME/CFS, arguing that it is due to inflammatory molecules entering the brain through opened sections of the BBB.[19] This process can continue for long periods and predispose a hypersensitive and over-active central nervous system, leading to further inflammatory and immune changes in the brain. The same I believe is true for long COVID.

For those reading this book who wish to know more about the science behind why the Perrin Technique™ helps long COVID, we need to look in more detail at some of the neuro-immune and physiological processes that become dysfunctional in this disorder. It is known that too much of one type of T-helper cell could potentially lead to autoimmune disease such as rheumatoid arthritis or chronic inflammatory states and cancer. This has led to scientists around the world viewing long COVID as an autoimmune disorder.[20]

A study by scientists in New York demonstrated that SARS-CoV-2 caused more permanent damage to the lung and kidney than the flu virus, impacting on the olfactory bulb and stimulating continuous T-cell activation and pro-inflammatory cytokine production even after a month following the acute phase of the infection.[21]

The body's immune system contains different types of cells, as described on page 173. Natural killer (NK) cells are important in the body's immune system, recognising and responding to infected cells. NK cells possess receptors allowing them to sense and respond to molecular patterns of bacteria, viruses, parasites and fungi, including 10 different types of protein. These NK receptors are known as 'toll-like receptors' (TLRs). They also react to certain environmental toxins.

It has been shown that high amounts of stress or a previous injury can predispose the TLRs to be more sensitive and release inflammatory molecules more readily in response to an immune stressor.[22] The reaction of the TLRs to the oxidative and nitrosative stress pathway leads to the production of more inflammatory molecules, which creates a vicious circle.[23, 24]

Also, a study looking into pathological changes in the lungs of COVID-19 victims showed interstitial fibrosis and revealed an abundance of inflammatory changes in the lung tissue. The autopsies also revealed major disruption and lesions in the spleen and surrounding lymph nodes.[25]

In long COVID this disturbance is not usually severe enough to stop the lungs and the lymphatic system functioning, but the damage often has a major effect on the quality of life.

The renin–angiotensin system (RAS)

Renin is an enzyme that is released into the circulation by the kidneys. Its release is stimulated by sympathetic nerve activation, reduction in blood pressure into the kidney, decreased salt transport within the kidney and an increase in prostaglandins in response to the reduced salt transport.

The brain renin–angiotensin system (RAS) works independently to the hormonal renin–angiotensin–aldosterone system (RAAS) and is involved in the regulation of water intake, salt appetite, blood pressure and autonomic functions. Up-regulation of angiotensin receptors in these nuclei has been shown to reduce baro-reflex sensitivity (that is, the speed with which signals from receptors in the aorta and carotid arteries control the brain's response to changes in blood pressure), and increase sympathetic tone, thus contributing to the development and maintenance of hypertension and heart failure.

As discussed in the previous chapter, this disturbed baro-reflex sensitivity explains why some patients with ME/CFS and FMS can also suffer from neurally-mediated hypotension and orthostatic intolerance and can also lead to the more severe condition known as POTS described on page 57.

When renin is released into the blood, it acts upon angiotensinogen to form angiotensin type 1. Angiotensin converting enzyme (ACE) is found in the walls of the blood vessels, especially in the lungs and heart, and transforms angiotensin 1 to angiotensin 2.

The main function of angiotensin 2 (ACE-2) is to cause the constriction of blood vessel walls, leading to increase in blood pressure. It also stimulates sodium reabsorption in the kidneys, increasing salt and water retention by the body.

It acts on the adrenal glands to release the hormone aldosterone, which also leads to increased sodium and fluid retention in the kidneys.

Angiotensin 2 stimulates the release of vasopressin (also known as antidiuretic hormone (ADH)) from the neurohypophysis – the posterior lobe of the pituitary gland – which increases fluid retention by the kidneys.

It also stimulates thirst centres within the brain and, most importantly in the pathogenesis of long COVID, it facilitates noradrenaline (norepinephrine) release from sympathetic nerve endings and inhibits noradrenaline re-uptake by nerve endings, thereby increasing the adrenaline-mediated function of the sympathetic nervous system. As we know, in most cases of long COVID we want to dampen the overstimulated sympathetic activity to help reduce symptoms and also improve neuro-lymphatic drainage.

Doctors prescribe 'ACE inhibitors', such as enalapril, fosinopril, lisinopril and ramipril, to help with blood pressure and cardiac problems, such as coronary artery disease. They are also often advised for diabetes, certain chronic kidney diseases and migraines.

The ACE inhibitors help relax the veins and arteries, leading to lower blood pressure. Side effects may include a dry cough, fatigue, dizziness from blood pressure going too low, headaches and loss of taste.

ACE inhibitors can also cause fluid retention in tissues, so basically one needs to maintain the correct balance of angiotensin 2 in the body to maintain the overall health of the cardiovascular and respiratory systems and much more.

Sometimes angiotensin receptor blockers (ARBs), such as losartan and telmisartan, are prescribed for cardiovascular disease, and sometimes aldosterone receptor blockers, such as spironolactone or eplerenone, have been helpful in heart and circulatory disorders.

Interestingly, it was shown that the coronavirus that caused SARS-CoV-1 in 2003 attached to ACE-2 receptors, especially in the lungs; plus, there is evidence that the SARS-CoV-2 related spike glycoprotein does the same.[26] COVID-19 patients treated with ACE inhibitors and ARBS have increased numbers of free ACE-2 receptors in their lungs.

As mentioned earlier, angiotensin acts on the posterior lobe of the pituitary gland, which is one of the circumventricular organs in the brain. Angiotensin also works on three more of these natural gaps in the BBB that make them vulnerable to infiltration by large toxins. These are the area postrema, the subfornical organ and the organum vasculosum, which have a critical role in maintaining blood pressure regulation and volume homeostasis via various nuclei located between the third ventricle and the brainstem.[27]

Acetylcholine-orchestrated neuromodulation in long COVID

Besides attaching to ACE-2 receptors. the spike protein also has a high affinity to nicotinic acetylcholine receptors which are the main structures in the cholinergic neuronal network responsible for autonomic, especially parasympathetic/vagal control. This connection has been demonstrated in a small study which saw long COVID patients' symptoms improve following the application of a nicotine patch.

Nicotine has a very high attraction to the receptors, 30 times more than acetylcholine, and therefore the application of a nicotine patch can displace the virus from these receptors, improving autonomic control, especially functioning of the vagus nerve.[28]

Before all my readers start applying nicotine patches, this was only a small study with just four patients tested. So, much more research is needed to validate the efficacy of nicotine in the arsenal against long COVID and rule out any serious side effects. It is also important to realise that the pathway blocked by the nicotine is only one of many sites in the body attacked by the SARS-CoV-2 coronavirus.

Predisposition to toxicity

Previous exposure to toxins will increase an individual's sensitivity to further toxic insult (attack). Some people have a greater genetic ability to detoxify while, unfortunately, others are more likely to experience more severe symptoms from toxic causes due to their individual genetic predisposition. Likewise, one's prior state of health, with the emphasis on the immune system, is a major significant factor to consider when assessing human ability to withstand exposure to poisonous chemicals. Age is important, with children much more susceptible to toxic overload than adults, because of their faster rate of absorption and smaller body weight – hence the smaller dosages of prescribed medicines allowed to children.[29]

Several chemicals have the potential to induce autoimmune diseases[30, 31, 32] such as systemic lupus erythematosus, commonly known as 'lupus' or 'SLE'.

Genetic susceptibilities have been discovered in diseases such as autoimmune hepatitis.[33] The immune profile and genetic predisposition in some long COVID sufferers is likely to render these individuals more prone to toxic attack. This has been termed 'ecogenetics'.[34] Also, let us not forget epigenetics, where gene expression can change due to external influences, such as increased toxins.

Important research is already taking place into genetic links with long COVID, such as a study by a UK research team which has already identified 73 genes associated with long COVID.[35]

Conclusion

We are all constantly bombarded by many poisons. One factor to sustain health is the ability to drain toxins away from body tissues, including the brain and spinal cord. If this drainage system is not working properly and/or pumping the fluid in the wrong direction, problems will arise, and if the neuro-lymphatic system becomes dysfunctional, neuro-immune illnesses such as long COVID will occur, increasing inflammation in the peripheral and central nervous systems and leading to dysfunction of many metabolic processes.

* Note relating to page 72: Magnetic spines and foreheads
Most toxic metals such as mercury are not very magnetic. However, if an electric current is passed through coils of metals surrounding a core of iron, a magnetic field is produced. A similar effect could occur if metals build up in the subcutaneous lymph vessels surrounding blood capillaries, which contain iron in haemoglobin – electric impulses from local nerves could create the magnetic phenomenon described. Indeed, I have already observed a stronger magnetic pull in the forehead and the upper thoracic spine when the patient's symptoms are more severe, indicating a corresponding larger build-up of metals in these areas.

Chapter 4

Treating long COVID using the Perrin Technique™

'I wish I could manage to be glad!' the Queen said. 'Only I never can remember the rule. You must be very happy, living in this wood, and being glad whenever you like!'

Alice Through the Looking Glass and What Alice Found There

Lewis Carroll

Case: Chloe's story

After the pandemic started in March 2020, like most people who had more time on their hands, I increased my exercise even more than normal. I was running 5 k up to three times a week and doing an hour of yoga daily. I've always enjoyed a busy lifestyle, seeing friends, going to festivals and living abroad – travelling here, there and everywhere. I also worked long hours in a career I loved, sometimes reaching 80 hours a week. I'd never had any health issues.

In September 2020 I tested positive for COVID. After a couple of weeks, I felt I had almost returned back to full health. I had a good amount of energy except I struggled with exercise. The day after even gentle yoga I had some joint and muscle pain, although I didn't think this was much to worry about at the time.

Then a couple of months after the initial infection I started a new job. With this increase in activity my symptoms worsened very quickly. Within three to four weeks I had wide ranging symptoms and was struggling to get out of bed. I visited the Perrin Clinic and received a diagnosis of long COVID. My sister had suffered from ME when we were younger and underwent the Perrin Technique™ with great results, so this was my first port of call as my symptoms seemed very similar.

I had debilitating fatigue and was now in bed the majority of the time. It was like waking up in the body of an 80-year-old and trying to figure out what the heck to do. I also suffered from heart palpitations, panic attacks, anxiety, brain fog, paranoia, sound sensitivity and insomnia, as well as general memory loss and confusion where I felt disorientated. I struggled to remember what I had done that morning, the day before or earlier in the week and in what order.

From my family's experience of the Perrin Technique™ I knew there was a good chance of recovery; however, I still struggled with acceptance of the situation. My life had completely changed in a matter of weeks. It was advised that I should stop working but I decided to continue with my new job remotely (most often from bed) whilst receiving the treatment. Because of this decision my recovery time has been much longer.

During the first few months of treatment I had some side effects. Initially my whole spine felt on fire from top to bottom and was sore. I often developed a rash over my back after the nightly massage. I had periods of vertigo. During the nasal drainage aspect of the self-treatment, I had a strong metallic taste at the back of my throat. My abdomen was also tender to touch, which Dr Perrin indicated was inflammation of the liver due to the toxins.

Over time I began to see improvements. I started to eat dinner together with my family rather than alone in my room and could have short phone conversations with friends. These may seem like small things but anyone suffering from long COVID knows these are important steps in the right direction. My anxiety slowly eased, and the panic attacks stopped.

Throughout the next couple of years all these small improvements have built up to mean I now live a full and healthy life, being able to live independently in my own flat once again. I am not yet 100% but I am very close! In the summer of 2023 I was finally able to enjoy a music festival with the support of my friends. I camped in a field and spent the days and nights dancing. It was a really big milestone and showed me how strong my body had become.

The people I had around me played a huge part in my recovery. My mum and sister would administer the at-home self-treatment daily and were very supportive, making sure I received as much care and rest as possible. This was instrumental in my recovery with the Perrin Technique™. I didn't spend time with people who weren't supportive of the condition and the treatment as I noticed that emotional stress was a key trigger. I saw an increase in symptoms following physical exertion but experienced far more impact after any emotional stress. It made me more careful and aware of stress at work and in my personal life as this can more easily be the cause of setbacks in my recovery.

I visited an NHS long COVID clinic during my recovery, mainly out of curiosity, where I was told there was nothing they could do for me except offer management techniques such as meditation. Although supportive, they offered no treatment plan. That's why I am so thankful for the Perrin Technique™ as without it I would likely have shown little to no improvement over the last few years. I am so grateful for Dr Perrin's knowledge and understanding of this condition – in addition to the treatment, he also provided answers at a distressing time.

Chloe McDonald, London.
Patient of Dr Raymond Perrin

History of the Perrin Technique™

My theory for the diagnosis and treatment of conditions such as long COVID started with one patient who had myalgic encephalomyelitis/chronic fatigue syndrome (ME/CFS).

In 1989 an executive, who shall be referred to as Mr E, walked into my city-centre practice, in Manchester, UK, where I ran a clinic specialising in the treatment of sports injuries. He had been a top cyclist, racing for one of the premier teams in the north-west of England. He had suffered from a recurring, low back pain, which, after examination, I had diagnosed to be a strain of the pelvic joints.

While treating his pelvis, I noted that the upper part of his back was particularly restricted. I enquired whether or not he had any prior problems in his upper back, and he acknowledged that for years, during his cycling, he had experienced a dull ache across his shoulders and at the top of his back. This in itself was nothing significant, as it was very common to find cyclists with pelvic problems and a stiff and disturbed curvature in the thoracic spine (the upper part of the backbone between the waist and the neck). What was interesting was the fact that, for the past seven years, Mr E had been diagnosed with ME/CFS. He complained of tingling in both hands and a 'muzzy' feeling in his head. He suffered general fatigue and an ache in his knees, as well as the pain in his back and shoulders. He had been forced to stop racing since the onset of the disorder. He was one of many patients who came to me after being diagnosed by their doctor, or specialist, as suffering from ME/CFS.

As I have said, he originally attended for treatment to his lower back. At that time, although I had helped other patients with ME/CFS, I had done no research into the disease, and I had no specific treatment programme for the disorder. With only five treatments, Mr E's back was better, but, most incredibly, the signs and symptoms of ME/CFS had dramatically improved. He was symptom-free after a mere two months from the start of treatment. After many years he continued to remain healthy and the last news I heard of him was that he had moved to Holland, cycling with the same power and zeal that he had used to enjoy prior to his illness.

It was after helping this patient that I realised that there must be a correlation between the mechanical strain on the thoracic spine and ME/CFS. Although I had not set out to help the fatigue signs and symptoms in this patient, I had done exactly that by improving his posture and increasing movement in his spine. My thoughts turned to the other ME/CFS patients that I had treated for back pain and biomechanical strain. The restriction of the dorsal spine was a common factor that could not be ignored. Since 1989, thousands of patients with signs and symptoms of ME/CFS have visited my clinic and also practices all over the world run by practitioners trained in the Perrin Technique™. None of them has presented with exactly the same symptoms but all have shared common structural and physical signs. This cannot be dismissed purely as coincidence.

The same symptoms have now been seen in long COVID patients by myself and my colleagues around the world. So, what is really going on? Below is a short recap of the theory underlying my technique and its relevance to long COVID which I have explained in some detail in Chapters 1–3.

Recap of lymphatic drainage and its role in ME/CFS and long COVID

Fact 1: Fluid flow

A fluid flows around the brain and continues up and down the spinal cord: this is the cerebrospinal fluid. This fluid has many functions – for example, as a protective buffer to the central nervous system and for supplying nutrients to the brain. However, one function has been discussed in osteopathic medicine since the 1860s but has received significant scientific attention only in recent years and that is the role it plays in the drainage of large molecules.

In fact, not only is there now visual evidence of the drainage system, but since I first published my theory, actual lymphatic vessels have been discovered in the membranes of the brain in both animal and human studies.

Fact 2: Getting the toxins out

The lymphatic system is an organisation of tubes around the body that provides a drainage system secondary to the blood flow. Why does the body need a secondary system to cope with poisons or foreign bodies in the tissues? Are the veins not good enough? The answer in one important word is 'size'. The blood does process poisons and particles, which enter the blood circulatory system via the walls of the microscopic blood vessels known as the capillaries. Their walls resemble a fine mesh which acts as a filter, thus allowing only small molecules to enter the bloodstream itself. When the blood reaches the liver, detoxification takes place, cleansing the blood of its impurities.

Larger molecules of toxins often need breaking down before entering the blood circulation, and they begin this process of detoxification in the lymph nodes on the way to drainage points just below the collar bone into two large veins (the subclavian veins), with most of the body's lymph draining into the left subclavian vein (see Fig. 8).

The capillary beds of lymphatic vessels, known as 'terminal' or 'initial lymphatics', take in any size of molecule via a wall that resembles the gills of a fish, opening as wide as is necessary to engulf the foreign body. The lymphatics also help to dispose of some toxins and impurities through the skin (via perspiration), urine, bowel movements and our breath. Once toxins have drained into the subclavian veins, they eventually find their way into the liver and, as is the case with normal circulatory toxins, are broken down by the liver.

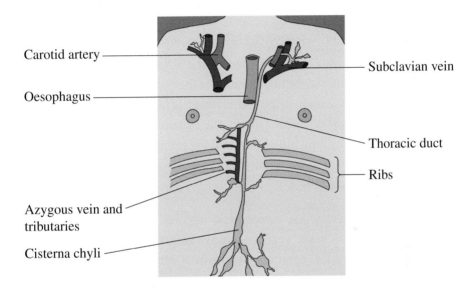

Fig. 8 The thoracic duct (the main central lymphatic drainage system into the blood).

Fact 3: The pumping mechanism

For over 300 years, from 1622 when Italian physician and anatomist Gasparo (Gaspere) Aselli (1581–1626) discovered the lymphatic system, it was thought not to have a pump of its own. Its flow was believed to depend on the massaging effect of the surrounding muscles and the blood vessels lying next to the lymphatics, akin to squeezing toothpaste out of a tube. However, we now know that the collecting vessels and ducts of the lymphatic system have smooth muscle walls, and Professor John Kinmonth, a London chest surgeon, discovered in the 1960s that the main drainage of the lymphatics, the thoracic duct, has a major pumping mechanism in its walls of around 4 beats a minute and that this is controlled by the sympathetic nervous system.[1, 2, 3, 4] If there is a disturbance of the sympathetic nervous system, the thoracic duct pumping mechanism may push the lymph fluid in the wrong direction and lead to a further build-up of toxins in the body.

Fact 4: The sympathetic nervous system

The sympathetic nervous system is part of the autonomic nervous system, which deals with all the automatic functions of the body. Although it is known for being the system which helps us in times of danger and stress, often referred to as the 'fight or flight' system, the sympathetic nervous system is also important in controlling blood flow and the normal functioning of all the organs of the body, such as the heart, kidneys and bowel. We know it is vital for healthy lymphatic drainage.

In long COVID sufferers, the sympathetic nervous system will have been placed under stress for many years before the infection of COVID-19. This stress may be of a physical nature due to postural strain or an old injury, or it may be emotional stress, or environmental stress, such as from pollution, or stress on the immune system due to infection or allergy.

The sympathetic nerves spread out from the thoracic spine to all parts of the body. The hypothalamus, just above the brain stem, acts as an integrator for autonomic functions, receiving regulatory input from other regions of the brain, especially the limbic system which involves emotion, motivation, learning and memory. Significantly, the hypothalamus also controls all the hormones of the body.

Fact 5: Biofeedback

The region of the brain called the hypothalamus controls hormones by a process called biofeedback. This mechanism can be explained with the following example. If the sugar levels in the body are too low, it may be due to a rise in the hormone insulin, which is produced in the pancreas, which lies in the upper right side of the abdomen beneath the liver. Insulin, like other hormones, is a large protein molecule that travels through the blood and stimulates the breakdown of sugar. It passes from the blood into the hypothalamus, which will calculate if more or less insulin production is required and, accordingly, send a message to the pancreas to make the necessary adjustments.

The region of the hypothalamus is one of a few sections of the brain that allow the transfer of large molecules into the brain from the blood. In all other parts of the brain there is a filter known as the blood–brain–barrier (BBB) allowing only small molecules to pass into the brain.

Unfortunately in many disease states, a damaged or disturbed BBB means that further large toxic molecules can invade the brain and wreak havoc on the normal functioning of the central nervous system, and in long COVID it has now been proven that many immune cells that promote inflammation do just that.[5]

Fact 6: What goes wrong?

The central nervous system, composed of the brain and the spinal cord, is the only region in the body that for hundreds of years was believed to have no true lymphatic system. Since we now know the lymphatics exist to drain large molecules, what can the central nervous system do if attacked by large toxins?

The lymphatic drainage of the central nervous system was actually first postulated as early as 1786 by Scottish military surgeon and chemist, William Cruikshank,[6] and a year later when the Italian anatomist Paolo Mascagni speculated that there were lymphatic vessels at the surface of the human brain.[7]

It has now been demonstrated that the cerebrospinal fluid (see Fact 1) drains toxins along minute gaps next to the blood along the brain and spinal cord's arterioles and venules known as para- and peri-vascular spaces (also known as Virchow-Robin spaces in the brain), and then into the lymphatic system outside the head through perforations in the skull and along spinal nerve pathways. The lymphatic vessels found in the head and around the spine take the toxins away via the thoracic duct and right lymphatic duct (see Fig. 8) into the blood and the liver where they are finally broken down.

This drainage mechanism in the brain has now been filmed in humans, with the largest amount draining through a bony plate (the cribriform plate) situated above the nose. The toxins then drain into lymphatic vessels in the tissue around the nasal sinuses. There is further drainage down the perivascular spaces supplying all of the other 12 pairs of cranial nerves, especially the ones in the eye (optic), ear (vestibulocochlear/acoustic) and cheek (trigeminal) respectively, and also down the spinal cord outwards to pockets of lymphatic vessels running alongside the spine.

This neuro-lymphatic drainage was termed 'the glymphatic system' in 2012 by Professor Maiken Nedergaard, Jeff Iliff and their colleagues at Rochester University in New York State after it was proven to exist in mice draining toxins from cells in the brain known as glia.[8] Glia are cells in the brain and nervous system generally that are not nerve cells (neurones) but support and feed nerve cells in a number of essential ways. The term means 'glue' as, until the 1970s, it was thought their only role was to hold nerve cells together. However, due to the pioneering work of London neurobiologist Professor Geoffrey Burnstock (1929–2020) we know that glial cells also have a major role in transmitting messages from one part of the brain to another via ATP.[9]

Glymphatic drainage has been shown to occur mostly during deep restorative sleep known as delta-wave sleep.[10] Many patients with long COVID complain that they don't get enough sleep and that, when they do, they still feel exhausted. The problem for them is that, although they may often have plenty of sleep, it isn't the restorative kind as it consists of a high proportion of shallow, non-restorative alpha-waves.

Researchers at Stanford University in the USA have shown that ME/CFS patients have fewer delta-waves during the night, but too many during the day.[11] The drainage of the brain and spinal cord occurs more during waking hours in ME/CFS and fibromyalgia (FMS), making those patients feel ill and shattered during the daytime. With long COVID, some patients have used wearable monitoring devices (such as FitBit or Garmin) to record that they are not having enough deep sleep either. Thus, during the night the brain switches on in long COVID patients (as in ME/CFS and FMS), leading to the 'tired but wired and fired' state, affecting most patients' ability to fall into a deep sleep which is when the restorative delta-wave sleep occurs, allowing the toxins to drain away from the brain.

Not only does the type of sleep affect glymphatic drainage, but it is the position a person adopts during sleep that is also vitally important. A side-lying posture during sleep aids neuro-lymphatic drainage,[12] as well as being the best position for the spine in general. Often, I am asked, 'Which side is best?' With regard to neuro-lymphatic drainage, I don't think it matters that much and I would advise you to start with lying on the side you feel most comfortable on. However, the left side is believed to be the better for improving venous return to the heart and also has been shown to reduce heartburn.

To maintain a balanced spine in bed, as well as lying on your side, I recommend a small pillow, such as a scatter cushion, placed between your knees throughout the night.

Fact 7: Build-up of toxins

In long COVID I believe it is these drainage pathways, in both the head and the spine, that are not working sufficiently, leading to a build-up of toxins within the central nervous system. The reasons for drainage problems can vary from patient to patient. It may be trauma to the head from a previous accident; it may be hereditary or due to a problem at birth. The spine may become out of alignment – especially in very active teenagers – which can lead to a disturbance in the normal drainage (see Fig. 9). If the spine and brain are both affected, the increased toxicity will disturb hypothalamic function and thus will further affect sympathetic control of the central lymphatic vessels. This in turn pumps more toxins back into the tissues and the brain, causing a vicious circle to ensue (see Fig. 10).

The neurotoxins described in detail in Chapter 3 may come in different shapes and sizes such as chemicals produced by ongoing emotional stress or environmental pollutants which are building up, usually for many years before the person is infected by COVID-19. However, in long COVID I believe, it is the massive production of large pro-inflammatory signalling proteins known as 'the cytokine storm' that is the probably the main triggering event.

New findings are emerging providing evidence for the build-up of inflammatory cytokines, such as interleukins IL-1β, IL-6 and tumour necrosing factor-alpha (TNF-α).[13]

Also found to be a major player is IL-1R2 leading to immune dysregulation in long COVID.[14] IL-1R2 is a particularly potent cytokine which has already been implicated in arthritis, endometriosis, diabetes, atherosclerosis, Alzheimer's disease and ulcerative colitis.[15]

The vicious circle that is shown in Fig. 10 results in the physical signs and symptoms described in detail in Chapter 2, including the frequent increase in temperature in the spine and upper abdomen from inflammatory toxins, varicose lymphatics, specific tender points, especially 'Perrin's Point', and tenderness of the solar plexus[16] – signs and symptoms that I have found in most of my long COVID patients since my first one in the early summer of 2020.[17] It also can result in a varied assortment of additional symptoms that are often dismissed by healthcare professionals as unrelated because the underlying mechanism that unites them is not understood.

Reducing inflammation

As we now know from the research studies mentioned above, there is a build-up of inflammatory proteins in long COVID. Therefore, the first task is to reduce

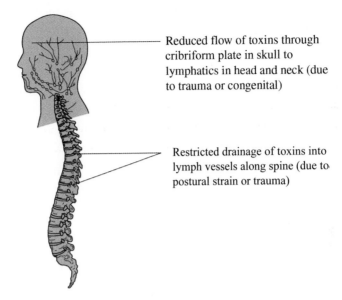

Fig. 9 Restricted drainage of toxins from the central nervous system.

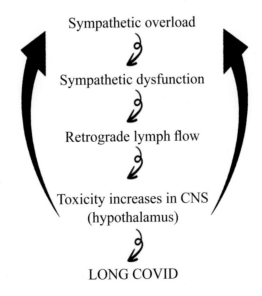

Fig. 10 The downward spiral into long COVID.

any possible inflammation present at the damaged segments of the spine. This can be achieved in various ways. Some practitioners would prescribe anti-inflammatory drugs. However, contrast bathing (warm alternating with cold) is deemed preferable, as it has no toxic side effects. The warm compress usually consists of a warm (not hot) water bottle. Too hot a compress could scald the patient's skin. The 'cold' is as cold as the patient can tolerate and this is sometimes just cool, i.e. fridge temperature; it is safer if a frozen pack is wrapped with a cover, especially as long COVID patients often cannot tolerate extremes of temperature. Frozen peas, which easily mould around the back, can also be used, although special cold compress packs, which remain soft even when frozen, are preferable and less messy, especially if the peas fall out of the bag!

My clinical experience has shown that the sequence of contrast bathing that gives the best results in reducing the inflammation in long COVID is as follows:

COLD	3 minutes	}
WARM	1 minute	}
COLD	1 minute	} Total 10 minutes
WARM	1 minute	}
COLD	1 minute	}
WARM	3 minutes	}

This process if done correctly has no adverse side effects, and so it is safe to be used as many times as required. Application at least three times a day to the upper thoracic region is recommended if there is inflammation in the neck and shoulders (or if there are cerebral symptoms such as brain fog – see Chapter 2), and to the lower thoracic area when the abdominal or lower extremities are affected. The main advantage of contrast bathing over anti-inflammatory drugs is that it works quickly and directly on the affected area. Even when there is no palpable or visible inflammation, shown by heat and redness, contrast bathing to improve circulation in the thoracic region is still advised as it will aid circulation in the region and improve sympathetic nerve activity which will, in turn, help the lymphatic drainage of the spine and improve the health of the tissue lying alongside the spine.

In July 2023 I presented a workshop at the International Association of CFS/ME conference held in Stony Brook University, Long Island, NY. The conference brought together leading scientists and clinicians from all corners of the world to discuss the latest breakthroughs in the field of ME/CFS, fibromyalgia and long COVID. There I met a wonderful scientist and author, Christopher Wikman from Maryland, USA. We spent many hours discussing our work and in appreciation, I gave him one of my books on ME/CFS.

After the conference was over he went back to his home and conducted a pilot study to examine the efficacy of using contrast bathing to improve sympathetic nerve activity. He used a computer-based NeuPT HRV Diagnostic System on a single subject and demonstrated an increase for heart rate variability (HRV) and health indices measured for the upper thoracic spinal region.

HRV is a measure of the variation in time between each heartbeat. This variation is controlled by the autonomic nervous system, with a higher HRV, or a wider variation of time intervals between heartbeats, indicating a balanced autonomic nervous system, showing that the body can adapt well to stress. This variable is increasingly used in physiological medicine to measure a person's overall wellness. A low HRV indicates that the sympathetic nervous system is dominant and overworking so to restore a balance one needs to increase the HRV.

Chris Wickman showed that over a five-week period of regular cold and warm compresses the thoracic health measures of the patient's HRV and other health indices, such as respiration and heart rates, overall improved by around 30%.

Long COVID patients who are suffering mostly from pain rather than fatigue may respond better to cold only on the spine for 5 minutes followed by, or at the same time, placing warm compresses or a warm water bottle on the surrounding muscles. For example, if there is much pain in the shoulders, arms and hands then the patient should apply warmth to these areas and the cold (not freezing) compress on the very bottom of the neck and upper back. This segment is known as the cervicothoracic or cervical-dorsal (CD) region of the spine; it is directly linked to a major bundle of sympathetic nerves known as the stellate ganglia, located at the level of C7, anterior to the transverse processes of C7 and the neck of the first ribs, just below the subclavian artery. Two of the main functions of the sympathetic nerves from the stellate ganglia are to control blood flow in the brain and also to stimulate the cardiac plexus, a network of autonomic nerve tissue responsible for innervating the cardiac tissue controlling the heart rate.

This region is so important that I warn Perrin Technique™ practitioners to be very gentle when treating this region and to avoid strenuous manipulation of the CD segment as it could easily overstimulate this region, disrupting the blood flow in the brain and disturbing the heart rate. Cold compresses at this region can help many patients with long COVID as this calms the sympathetic nerves in this region.

Two long COVID patients found relief following stellate ganglion blocking with the use of a local anaesthetic.[18] However, one can help without any invasive treatment, by simply pressing a cool compress (not freezing) a few times a day for around 5 minutes on the CD region.

If the pain is in the legs and feet, then warm these areas and at the same time place cool packs on the upper lumbar spine, around the waist level. This is the level supplying the bottom of the sympathetic nerve chains mentioned earlier and this process will hopefully reduce the overstimulation of the sympathetic nerves of the abdomen, legs and feet.

Treating long COVID using the Perrin Technique™

How osteopathy helps

The Perrin Technique™ is primarily an osteopathic technique. Many of you reading this book may be more familiar with COVID-19 and long COVID than with osteopathy. By now you may have a clearer understanding of the biophysical processes leading to the susceptibility of developing a post-viral syndrome, but you may still be wondering how osteopathy can help.

One of the major concepts of osteopathy is that the structure of the body governs the function of the organs within. Osteopaths work on the principle that a patient's history of illnesses and physical traumas is written into the body's structure. It is the osteopath's developed sense of touch (palpatory sense) that enables the practitioner manually to diagnose while treating the patient. The osteopath's job is to restore a healthy structure to the body and thereby its function. The osteopath gently applies manual techniques of massage and manipulation to encourage movement of the bodily fluids, eliminate dysfunction in the motion of the tissues, relax muscular tension and release compressed bones and joints. The areas being treated require proper positioning to assist the body's ability to regain normal tissue function. Osteopathy was officially established on 22 June 1874 and as I finish writing this book our profession has just celebrated its 150th birthday. One of the key principles of our profession laid down by its founder, Dr Andrew Taylor Still (1828–1917), is that illness is mainly due to stagnation of body fluids and that if you can stimulate blood flow and other fluid motion, including cerebrospinal fluid and lymphatic drainage, then the body will recover.

One of AT Still's students, William Garner Sutherland (already mentioned on page 38), noticed that when the bones of a dis-articulated skull were viewed in a certain way, they resembled the gills of a fish. Accordingly, he hypothesised, in 1898, that their shape was designed to allow for movement and so cranial osteopathy was born. By gentle pressure on the head one can help this movement aid the lymphatic drainage of the brain; as Sutherland said: 'When

103

you tap the waters of the brain see what happens in the lymphatic system.'

Lubrication for effleurage

Congested and varicose lymphatics throughout the body are relieved by 'effleurage', a method of massage that requires stroking motions along the surface of the head, neck and trunk. To avoid any friction, which will aggravate any inflammatory condition, practitioners and patients must use plenty of lubrication when carrying out the effleurage. The type of oil or cream is very important. It should be hypo-allergenic and unscented. The oils that I use are coconut oil and sweet almond oil, although some practitioners prefer using an aqueous cream. Baby oil is not suitable, as it is a perfumed mineral oil, a by-product of refining crude oil used to make gasoline and other petroleum products.

The main focus of the treatment is to massage the lymph always in the direction towards the collar bones in a technique that I call the 'concertina effect' (see below). As in a concertina or an accordion, where putting pressure on the ends of the bellows forces air through the instrument to produce the desired musical effect, so effleurage performed towards either clavicle (collarbone) on both sides creates a pressure that forces the lymph to drain out through the central drainage system into the subclavian veins (see Fig. 1, page 29). This increased pressure of lymphatic fluid produced within the lymphatic ducts creates a negative pressure in the lymphatic vessels above and below, which then produces an action similar to what is known as the 'siphon effect'; this is familiar to anyone who has ever cleaned out the bottom of a fish tank – sucking on a tube creates a pressure gradient. Fluid will always flow from an area under higher pressure to an area of lower pressure. So, lymph will continue to drain from the entire system, eventually including the lymphatic system of the brain and spinal cord. Toxins stuck in the central nervous system, some for many years, will slowly and surely drain away after being sucked up, just like the siphon tube in the fish tank, into the main trunks and ducts of the lymphatic system.

The osteopathic techniques that I have developed to treat ME/CFS, FMS and now long COVID patients are based on some new procedures that I have developed, but mainly on adapted standard procedures used by osteopathic practitioners and some physiotherapists and chiropractors and other manual therapists.

Some of the methods of treatment mentioned in this chapter are more directed to the practitioner, but most patients want to know what the treatment entails so the next section will describe the processes and procedures that make up the Perrin Technique™ plus other manual techniques that may be employed by the practitioner to help improve the patient's biomechanical health.

The 10 steps of the Perrin Technique™

The manual treatment of each long COVID patient (preferably performed by a licensed Perrin Technique™ practitioner) consists of the following 10 steps or stages:

1. Effleurage to aid drainage in the breast tissue lymphatics
2. Effleurage to aid drainage in the cervical lymphatic vessels
3. Gentle articulation of the thoracic region and soft tissue techniques with upward effleurage
4. Effleurage to aid drainage in the cervical lymphatic vessels
5. Soft tissue massage to relax muscles and encourage lymph drainage of the cervico-thoracic region
6. Further cervical effleurage towards the subclavian region
7. Functional and inhibition techniques to the suboccipital region
8. Further cervical effleurage towards the subclavian region
9. Stimulation of the cranio-sacral rhythm by cranial and sacral techniques
10. Final cervical effleurage towards the subclavian region.

As Rudyard Kipling (1865–1936) once said: 'The cure for this ill is not to sit still.' Movement is an essential part of the healing process. So, gentle exercises are prescribed to improve the quality of thoracic spine mobility and the coordination of the patient. The treatment schedule listed above is almost the same as the protocol followed throughout clinical trials for ME/CFS that my colleagues and I conducted in the years 1996–1997 and 2000–2001. It has altered slightly over the years as I have found that certain techniques further improve the neuro-lymphatic drainage. The amount of time spent, and the pressure exerted on to the patient whilst using these techniques, depends on the physical state of the patient and on the symptom picture at that particular stage in their treatment. So, as always with long COVID, every patient requires distinctly specific techniques with individual treatment sessions marginally different from each other.

Step 1: Effleurage to aid drainage in the breast tissue lymphatics

The gentle strokes of effleurage are carried out rhythmically towards the subclavian region, at the level of the left and right subclavian veins, which drain all the lymph fluid into the bloodstream. Effleurage stimulates the lymphatic drainage through direct routes into the thoracic duct and the right lymphatic duct and hence into the venous return (see Fig. 11). Care is taken to avoid stimulating drainage into the axillary lymph nodes in the armpit, which are prone to swelling and congestion in long COVID sufferers due to the backflow of lymph. It is hypothesised that the more direct route forces a high pressure within the smaller parasternal vessels, which creates enough force within the thoracic duct to alleviate the backpressure and restore a healthy drainage of toxins into the venous return.

When male practitioners are treating female patients, effleurage to the breast tissue should be carried out in the presence of a chaperone, if one is available, after explaining the exact nature of the treatment and using consent forms usually supplied by the practitioner's governing body. The gentle stroking is applied upwards covering the entire breast tissue towards the clavicle using the backs of the hands so not to be too heavy-handed. Also, the back of the hand offers a less invasive approach.

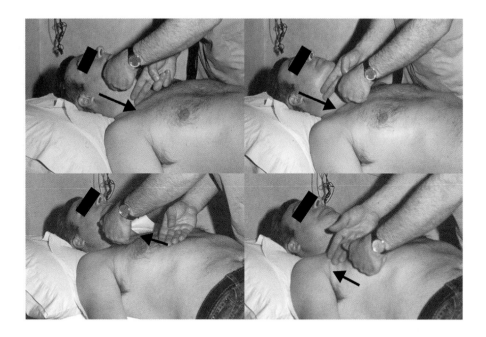

Fig. 11. Effleurage down neck and up chest to clavicle.

Step 2: Effleurage to aid drainage in the cervical lymphatic vessels

After pushing the lymph upward in the chest, it is followed by further effleurage down the front and sides of the neck towards the clavicle remembering to use lots of oil to reduce friction.

The black arrows in Fig. 11 show the direction of the massage technique, which is always towards either clavicle on both sides. This is the region above the drainage of lymphatic fluid from the right lymphatic duct and the thoracic duct into the right and left subclavian veins respectively.

The concertina and siphon effect

This continual massage towards the subclavian region creates what I call 'the concertina effect' as described above. As in a concertina or an accordion, where putting pressure on the ends of the bellows forces air through the instrument to produce the desired musical effect (see Fig. 12), so effleurage performed towards either clavicle on both sides creates a pressure that forces the lymph to drain out through the central drainage into the subclavian veins (see Fig. 13).

This increased pressure of lymphatic fluid produced within the thoracic and right lymphatic ducts creates a negative pressure in the lymphatic vessels

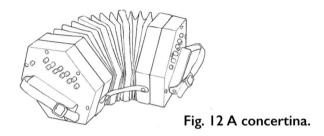

Fig. 12 A concertina.

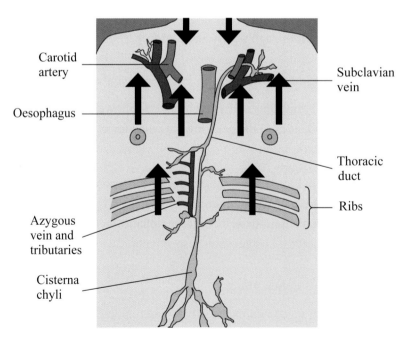

Carotid artery

Subclavian vein

Oesophagus

Thoracic duct

Ribs

Azygous vein and tributaries

Cisterna chyli

Fig. 13 The concertina effect.

above and below, which then produces the siphon effect described earlier in this chapter. As I noted, fluid will always flow from an area under higher pressure to an area under lower pressure. So, lymph will continue to drain from the entire system, eventually including the lymphatic system of the brain and spinal cord. Toxins stuck in the central nervous system, some for many years, will slowly and surely drain away after being sucked up.

Step 3: Gentle articulation of the thoracic region and soft tissue techniques with upward effleurage

The next step is gentle articulation of the thoracic and upper lumbar spine, plus long-lever stretching and articulation of the ribs along with longitudinal soft tissue stretching plus effleurage of the paraspinal lymphatic vessels – the lymphatics that run up either side of the spine.

This combination of gentle articulation and soft tissue techniques improves movement of the thoracic and upper lumbar spine plus the ribs and relaxes the paravertebral muscles, trapezii, levator scapulae, rhomboids and muscles of respiration. This is achieved together with the upward effleurage from the waist to the level of the collarbone to increase the lymphatic drainage of the spine.

The main objective of the articulatory, soft tissue techniques and occasional high velocity manipulation is to improve the structure and overall quality of movement of the dorsal and upper lumbar spine.

All the articulatory techniques are slowly and gently applied with minimal force in order to avoid irritating spinal inflammation and to reduce any reactive spasm from the surrounding muscles.

The two sympathetic nerve trunks are integrally related to the overall structure of the area. By reducing mechanical irritation at this region, as well as relaxing disturbed afferent impulses, the dysfunction of the sympathetic nervous system can be corrected. There are perivascular spaces along the nerves that enter and leave the spinal cord. Improving the biomechanics of the spine and lymphatic flow in this region aids overall neuro-lymphatic drainage. This is all helped by the very rhythmic and gentle nature of this technique, which, when combined with stretching and movement of the ribs, creates an extremely relaxing yet powerful treatment, not just for long COVID, but also for many upper body mechanical dysfunctions and general back pain.

If starting lower than the thoracic spine, i.e. on the upper lumbar region, this technique will also help relax the crura of the diaphragm – the muscular wall between the abdomen and thorax. The crura are the two tendinous structures that join the diaphragm to the upper lumbar vertebrae. The thoracic duct, the central 'drainage pipe' of the lymphatics, passes through the diaphragm alongside the largest artery, the aorta. Helping to reduce diaphragmatic tension will aid lymphatic drainage. To quote the founder of osteopathy, Andrew Taylor Still: 'At this point I will draw your attention to what I consider is the cause of a whole list of hitherto unexplained diseases, which are only effects of the blood and other fluids being prohibited from doing normal service by constrictions at the various openings of the diaphragm. Thus, prohibition of the free action of the thoracic duct would produce congestion.'[19]

In cases of hypermobility, which is rarely found in a patient's thoracic spine, mobility of the adjoining areas of the spine is improved by articulation and manipulation. This takes the strain off the hypermobile segments. What is predominantly found in patients with long COVID, as I have said repeatedly, is a restricted dorsal spine. Frequently, the entire thoracic region is stiff, while occasionally just a few segments are affected. However, one of the most common mechanical disturbances seen in long COVID is a mid-thoracic spine that is flatter and more rigid than normal. Together with the mid-thoracic problem that most commonly affects T4, T5 and T6 segments, is the hypermobility of the upper cervical and the lower lumbar regions – in other words, the very top and bottom of the mobile spinal column.

This step of the treatment is carried out with the patient lying on their side to allow a gentle stretch of periscapular and paravertebral muscles together with gentle massage upwards along the spine to improve lymphatic flow. This is combined with a gentle stretch of the ribs, which is performed by holding the patient's arm with one hand whilst massaging up the angles of the ribs near the vertebrae with the other, and gently moving the held arm upwards, stretching the diaphragm and thorax. Combined stretch and massage, using the patient's arm as a long lever, produces excellent results, with movement of the ribs increased by articulatory stretch techniques (see Fig. 14).

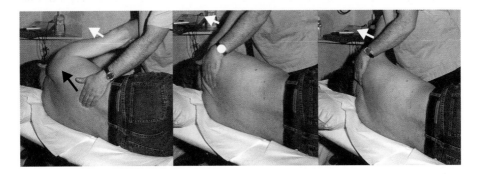

Fig. 14 Combined articulation, soft tissue stretches and paraspinal effleurage.

Generally, the massage technique for the relaxation of all the paraspinal muscle groups takes the form of gentle but deep longitudinal upward strokes with the hypothenar eminence of the practitioner's hand. This is the bulge of the palm formed by the three muscles that help control the little finger. With the massaging hand slightly cupped, the practitioner should use a tad more pressure from the pads of their fingers to drain the paraspinal lymphatics up towards the central drainage into the blood at the level of the first thoracic vertebra. Care should be taken to carry out this effleurage technique without pressing on the spinous processes to avoid irritating the inflamed spine. When treating long COVID patients with fibromyalgia-type symptoms, where severe widespread pain is the dominant complaint, one should do less soft tissue massage and carry out more of the long lever stretching techniques.

Besides stretching, I occasionally use more specialised osteopathic methods known as inhibition or functional techniques, which involve gentle pressure or positional holds. These are used to reduce the tone of the tightened musculature, especially of the diaphragm itself, known as 'diaphragmatic release', as described below.

Fig. 14 shows the combination of three soft tissue techniques: long lever stretches of the intercostal muscles, using the patient's arm as a lever; direct longitudinal stretch of the dorsal erector spinae with the cupped hand; and effleurage to the paravertebral lymphatics using the fingertips. The black arrow illustrates the direction of the massage, and the white arrows show the direction of movement of the patient's arm.

I try to avoid lying the patient in a prone position to avoid unnecessary pressure on the breast tissue. However, if the practitioner finds it necessary for the patient to lie prone, their face should be placed into a breathing hole in the treatment plinth to avoid unnecessary strain on the neck. The patient should be positioned on to their side as soon as possible, in order to carry out the paravertebral soft tissue work in this healthier position, while keeping the head horizontal and level, with the knees apart with the aid of pillows.

After increasing the movement of the restricted spine and relaxing the surrounding musculature, an attempt to improve the respiratory mechanics is undertaken. This is important in long COVID patients, since the amount of oxygen in the body affects the chemical content of the body and this has a direct effect on the functioning of the body's tissues. Reduced oxygen produces greater fatigue in the patient and will aggravate the symptoms. By improving the mechanics of respiration in the rib cage, the patient's lung capacity is increased during inspiration (breathing in), thus raising the patient's oxygen intake. Inspiration has been shown to aid cerebrospinal fluid motion, which in turn aids the cranial rhythmic impulse which I believe drives neuro-lymphatic drainage, as explained later in this section (Step 9).[20]

Although increasing spinal mobility and relaxing paravertebral muscles will enhance movement of the ribs, the specific respiratory muscles should also be treated in order to improve respiratory mechanics. These include the intercostal muscles, serratus anterior and posterior, pectorals, abdominals and, most importantly, the diaphragm. As stated above, gentle inhibition to the edge of the diaphragm dome – diaphragmatic release – will usually reduce the tone of the muscle and aid breathing.

After increasing the mobility of the thorax by articulation and stretching, as well as relaxing the musculature, the patient usually feels more comfortable and can lie in a supine position with knees slightly bent in readiness for the next step of the treatment.

Step 4: Effleurage to aid drainage in the cervical lymphatic vessels

After pushing the lymph upwards in the back, it is again followed by further effleurage down the front and sides of the neck towards the clavicle, again creating the concertina effect, remembering to use lots of oil/aqueous cream to reduce friction.

Step 5: Soft tissue massage to relax muscles and encourage lymph drainage of the cervico-thoracic region

The next step of the treatment is to relax the trapezii levator scapulae and periscapular muscles – for example, the rhomboids, as well as any other hypertonic back, shoulder and lower neck muscles (see Fig. 15).

As with the other muscular stretching techniques, this 'kneading' of the trapezii and associated shoulder and cervical muscles should always be towards the sub-clavicular region in the front, level with the first thoracic vertebra in the back (see Fig. 15). This is combined with a kneading technique that also incorporates gentle effleurage of the surface lymphatics towards the clavicles.

Many practitioners find this step of the technique challenging since many physios and osteopaths are originally taught to massage the muscles of the neck upwards when carrying out kneading techniques of the trapezii. This is plainly wrong as it ignores the direction of lymph towards the subclavicular veins beneath the collar bones.

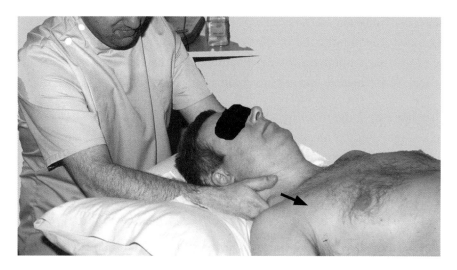

**Fig. 15 Longitudinal and cross fibre stretching of
lower neck and shoulders (trapezii and levator scapulae muscles).**

This technique involves a slow rhythmic kneading action applied across the
fibres of the lower cervical erector spinae, trapezii and levator scapulae with
gentle downward effleurage with the thumbs superficially along the border of
the sternocleidomastoid muscles using plenty of oil to avoid any friction.

Step 6: Further cervical effleurage towards the subclavian region

After pushing the lymph downwards in the front, it is again followed by
further effleurage down the front and sides of the neck using the backs of
your fingers downwards towards the clavicle, remembering to use lots of oil
to reduce friction.

Step 7: Functional and inhibition techniques to the suboccipital region

Two major regions that often require attention when dealing with spinal
problems are the suboccipital region, where the upper neck meets the cranium,
and the lumbosacral area which is where the lumbar spine joins to the wedge-

shaped bone at its base, the sacrum. It is important when one treats posturo-mechanical strain of the spine to balance the suboccipital and lumbosacral segments. Any abnormal curvature will alter muscle tone along the spinal column and thus place extra load on the uppermost section and base of the spine. Similarly, positional alterations at the top and bottom of the spinal column will affect the overall mechanics of the entire spine.

Osteopaths and chiropractors may use an effective procedure in these regions known as the functional technique (see Fig. 16). If, during subtle movement of the spine, a restriction is detected, however slight, the back is held at the point of restriction until a release of muscle tension occurs. In practice, osteopaths rely on finely developed palpatory skills. The main principle of any osteopathic treatment is that structure governs function. The principle of the functional technique is that, by placing a joint or a group of muscles in a certain position that is functionally suited for that particular bodily part, the result is a relaxation of tissues and an overall improvement in muscular and fascial tone in the region.

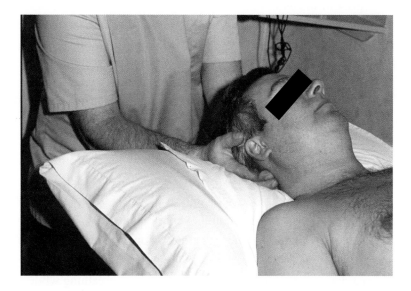

Fig. 16 Functional technique to the suboccipital region.

The suboccipital muscles can be relaxed efficiently and painlessly using this technique. With the patient lying supine (on their back), the osteopath's hands are placed at each side cradling the occiput, which is then lifted slightly off the pillow. The cervical spine is then gently extended and slowly rotated and bent towards the right or left. Traction or compression is applied and, by asking the patient to breathe deeply, one is able to utilise exhalation as a relaxation tool.

A further technique that I often employ to reduce the tone in the suboccipital muscles is known as 'inhibition'. This involves the patient lying supine with the practitioner cradling the back of the patient's head. Gentle pressure is then exerted through the practitioner's finger tips just below the base of the skull and held in a fixed position, and as the pressure increases to a certain level specific to each individual case, the skilled practitioner should feel the tightness in the tone of the muscles slowly and surely 'melt' away. This technique can lead to a significant relaxation of the offending musculature.

The occipito–atlantial joint is the joint between the top vertebra of the neck, the atlas, and the back of the skull, the occiput. This joint is extremely important for the integrity of the autonomic nervous system as is the atlanto–axial joint (the joint below the atlas with the second cervical vertebra, the axis). In fact, if there is any problem with this region of the spine, many severe symptoms can arise. This is because of two main factors:

1. The Xth cranial nerve, the vagus, leaves the cranium and travels out of the spine in this region. If it were to be irritated, as has been discussed in Chapter 3, it could affect many of the body's functions, especially the heart rate and the digestive system. As we now know from the work of Dr Steven Porges, there are two distinct parts of the vagus: the ventral vagus at the front and the dorsal vagus at the back. Trauma and irritation in the cranio-vertebral region could overstimulate the dorsal vagus which can lead to worsening of some symptoms, slowing down the metabolism to a pathological level, leading to symptoms such as slow heart rate (bradycardia) and sleep apnoea when one can stop breathing while asleep.

2. The vertebral arteries. There are two major arteries travelling up each side

of the cervical spine. These vertebral arteries enter the cranium alongside the spinal cord and if there is a mechanical problem this can affect the flow to the brain.

Major injury to either of the vertebral arteries is rare; however, if the flow along the artery is impaired by possible arthritic changes in the cervical spine or postural and mechanical strain to the neck, it may lead to a condition known as vertebral artery insufficiency which can cause dizziness and other neurological injury, but often the symptom is head and suboccipital (uppermost region of the neck) pain. It can occur following severe trauma, but it is more common due to wear and tear of the region.

One of the leading pioneers of integrative medicine, Dr Mosaraf Ali, stresses the importance of a good flow of the vertebral arteries in his book *The Neck Connection*. As Dr Ali maintains, the carotid arteries at the front of the neck are only found in mammals and supply blood to the conscious brain. The vertebral arteries found in all vertebrates supply blood to the subconscious part of the brain, including the hypothalamus and the other centres of the autonomic nervous system. Dr Ali, although not an osteopath or chiropractor, holds by osteopathic and chiropractic principles that problems around the spine can lead to many disorders. In the neck, mechanical problems can lead to psychological and emotional as well as physical symptoms. By improving the structure and function of the cervical vertebrae one can help the cerebral blood flow, restoring overall health to the central nervous system and the whole body.[21]

As mentioned previously, many patients who develop long COVID have injured their heads in the past. A trauma to the cranium, especially the top of the head, may result in a compression injury causing restriction of the suboccipital region. However, as discussed in Chapter 6, hypermobility in this region is common in some serious cases where patients may also have Ehlers-Danlos hypermobility type syndrome (see comorbidities in Chapter 2, page 53). There is a group of long COVID patients who also exhibit extreme symptoms, which worsen on extension of this region, which could very well be due to a Chiari malformation, as discussed in Chapter 2. The most serious cases of cranio-cervical instability require surgery to fuse the bones and stabilise the joint. However, most can be helped with the correct gentle strengthening exercises detailed in the self-help section found later in Chapter 7 (page 195).

Step 8: Further cervical effleurage towards the subclavian region

After working on the suboccipital region, once again the practitioner should carry out further effleurage down the front and sides of the neck towards the clavicle.

Step 9: Stimulation of the cranio-sacral rhythm by cranial and sacral techniques

Cranial stimulation commences near the end of each consultation (see Fig. 17). This technique is the most important and powerful part of the treatment as it directly affects the fluctuating, slow-wave previously described by Sutherland,[22, 23] known as the cranial rhythmic impulse (CRI), which, according to my hypothesis, is the pulse of neuro-lymphatic drainage. Cranial techniques have been shown to be effective in helping all aspects of the patient's health.

In this technique, the osteopath's hand is placed in two different positions, cradling the head laterally and antero-posteriorly. The cranial procedure involves very gentle pressure and minimal movements. The CRI has a flexion (inspiration) phase and an extension (expiration) phase, faintly changing the shape of the ventricles. Similar to the effects of the thoracic duct pump influencing the entire lymphatic system, the CRI can, by skilled practitioners, be palpated throughout the body as the lymph spreads throughout the organs and limbs. Added to that, retired plastic surgeon Dr Joel Pessa has demonstrated that the drainage of cerebrospinal fluid from the central nervous system continues alongside peripheral nerves throughout the body.[24]

The main cranial technique I use is a procedure known in the osteopathic world as the Sutherland or vault hold. Most osteopaths use a technique known

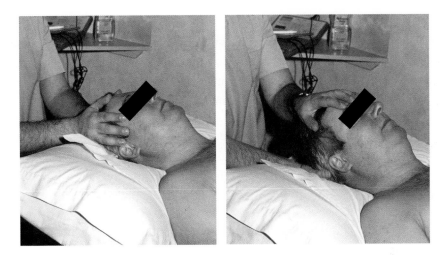

Fig. 17 Cranial treatment.

as CV4 (the compression of the fourth ventricle), although I believe it does effect a compression to the ventricular system as a whole.

In both these holds, the compression is achieved by gentle force applied with both hands, pressing medially at the lateral angles of the occiput and around the side of the head. This is followed by rhythmically expanding the cranium by gently opening the hands and lifting the pressure of the cranium. The direction of force through the hands and arms of the practitioner when applying this technique resembles the mechanism of pumping and sucking the air in and out of a blacksmith's bellows but with far less pressure and amplitude (see Fig. 18).

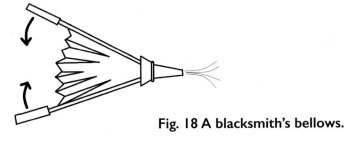

Fig. 18 A blacksmith's bellows.

During the compression phase of this gentle technique, the volume within the ventricular system is reduced, forcing the cerebrospinal fluid out. Thus drainage through the olfactory, optic, trigeminal and auditory pathways plus down the spine is enhanced and accordingly, by directly improving the neuro-lymphatic drainage, it plays an important part in overall treatment.

The vault hold and the CV4 have both recently been shown in scientific studies to help balance the autonomic nervous system, providing further evidence to support my hypothesis that the CRI is produced by the neuro-lymphatic drainage mechanism improving the function of the hypothalamus.[25, 26]

The other main cranial hold which achieves a similar effect is known as the occipito–frontal hold, again cradling the occiput, but this time in the centre of the rear of the skull, with one hand underneath the cranium and the other hand gently pressing down in the centre of the patient's forehead.

Although to the observer, and indeed from the patient's point of view, cranial techniques may look very gentle, they are extremely powerful and often produce major changes with only a little application There are more specialised cranial techniques that I sometimes use and this is all about the individuality of the treatment, palpating the patient's specific needs at the time of each treatment, so the holds may vary at each treatment, regarding how long and how much pressure one uses. Generally, it is very gentle, with the patient feeling very little going on until the cranial treatment is over. Cranial techniques, however, should always be done after the previous eight steps of the technique mentioned above.

Some practitioners refer to the CRI as the cranio–sacral rhythm. This is due to the fact that the rhythm can be palpated easily at the sacrum at the base of the spine as the cerebrospinal fluid moves down the spine from the cranium to the sacrum and then turns back and up towards the brain. The practitioner can palpate and further stimulate the CRI at this level by cradling the sacral bones when the patient lies supine (face up) (see Fig. 19).

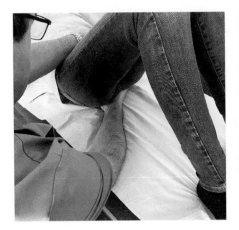 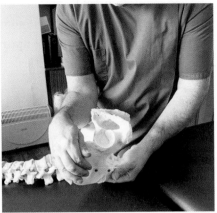

Fig. 19 Sacral treatment.

One of the osteopath's hands is held under the sacrum while the other hand balances the pelvic girdle from the front making very slight postural changes to the region. These minute changes due to altered direction of pressure from both hands allow subtle changes in the cerebrospinal fluid mechanism that can have major effects on the neuro-lymphatics and the overall spinal neural pathways.

Step 10: Final cervical effleurage towards the subclavian region

The treatment is completed by a final few seconds of effleurage down the front and sides of the neck towards the clavicle.

Manual procedures additional to the Perrin Technique™

On top of the 10-step treatment protocol, the practitioner will occasionally need to employ other techniques that are not taught in the standard Perrin Technique™ training but are useful for some patients in certain circumstances. These include high velocity–low amplitude manipulation of the thoracic and upper lumbar spinal segments using supine and side-lying combined leverage and thrust techniques. Also, sometimes the diaphragm is very tight under the ribs and requires direct techniques to relax this important muscle. **NB. Not all practitioners are trained to use some of these techniques so it is important that the patient seeks out the appropriate practitioner who may wish to employ some of these modalities.**

The sequence, strength and duration of all the above techniques are based on each individual case, but practitioners should take care not to over-manipulate, especially in the lower cervical region, as this can severely exacerbate the symptoms… remember: 'Less is more'.

High velocity–low amplitude manipulation ('clicketypops')

These techniques are generally taught in osteopathic, chiropractic and some physiotherapy colleges. If any of the joints are severely immobile, it may prove necessary to increase movement (see Figs 20, 21 and 22). In osteopathy, this technique is called high velocity–low amplitude (HVLA) or simply the high velocity thrust (HVT). In chiropractic, this manoeuvre is called an 'adjustment' and is commonly known as a manipulation. Physiotherapists call it 'Maitland mobilisation grade 5'.

This manoeuvre is the best-known technique in the osteopath's armoury and involves a short, sharp motion usually applied to the spine. This procedure is designed to release structures with a restricted range of movement. There are various methods of delivering a high velocity thrust. Chiropractors are more likely to push on vertebrae with their hands, whereas osteopaths tend to use the limbs to make levered thrusts. That said, osteopathy, hands-on physiotherapy and chiropractic techniques are converging, and much of their therapeutic repertoire is shared. This technique may produce a 'cracking' sound. For my younger patients, I reduce the anxiety concerning this technique by referring to it as 'clicketypops' treatment which usually brings a smile to the young patients and their parents' faces.

The HVTs of the thoracic spine can be achieved with the patient lying prone (on their front), but it is preferable and safer to turn the patient on to their back and manipulate them in a supine position. Vertebral joints in some patients may appear slightly fused, and therefore strong manipulation should be avoided in order to prevent any damage to the bone.

In Fig. 20, my left hand is positioned in a loose fist around the spinous process of the vertebra. As pressure is exerted from my right hand downwards, the force directed along the plane of the facet joints at the side of adjacent vertebrae will cause this joint between the vertebrae to gap. When the tension has built up by positioning the patient's upper spine in a flexed and rotated position, a fast but gentle pressure is applied through the direction of force as illustrated by the arrow which further gaps the joint and brings about a long-lasting increase in mobility.

In Fig. 21, the upper lumbar vertebrae are gently rotated, creating tension at a restricted joint. By applying a further quick thrust with my hands across the joint it opens and creates more overall movement.

Fig. 22 shows this manipulative procedure, which involves bending the patient's neck to the left while rotating the cervical spine towards the right. Gentle pressure is placed towards the direction of the arrow, gapping the joints at the side of the restricted vertebrae, creating more movement.

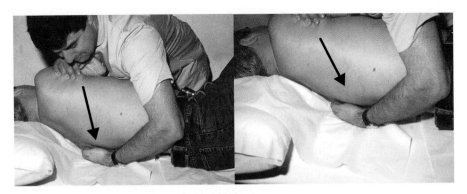

Fig. 20 Combined leverage and thrust of mid-thoracic vertebrae.

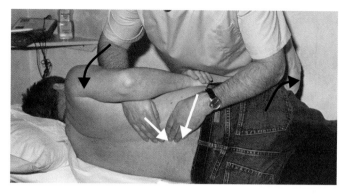

Fig. 21 Combined leverage and thrust on the upper lumbar spine.

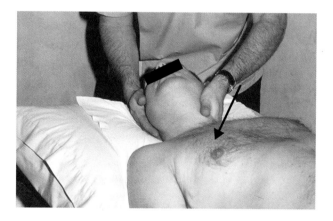

Fig. 22 Gentle combined leverage and thrust on the lower cervical spine.

Functional techniques on the sacrum and the pelvic and lower lumbar spine

Similar to the functional technique to the suboccipital region of the neck, with the patient lying supine, gentle movements are applied to the pelvic and lower lumbar region by cradling one hand under the patient's sacrum and palpating the muscle tone in the lumbar-sacral region. Traction or compression is applied and, by asking the patient to breathe deeply, one is able to utilise exhalation as a relaxation tool. There is a fixed position where, by palpating the muscle tone in the lower lumbar region just above the sacrum, one is able to feel the point of maximum relaxation for the pelvic and lumbar erector spinae muscles. As with other functional techniques, this position is held for a short period, resulting in a reduction of tone in this muscle group.

Inhibition and functional techniques only take a few minutes to achieve their effects, so are excellent extra tools to use alongside the standard treatment protocol of the Perrin Technique™.

Intra-oral cranial

There are more direct techniques to the cranium such as intra-oral techniques, which involve the practitioner using their fingers to open up the cribriform plate drainage from underneath by applying pressure on certain parts of the hard palate (with gloves on, of course). However, I urge caution about using such direct techniques in the early stages of treatment as it could result in too much toxic drainage through the olfactory pathway leading to a crash of the patient's symptoms. So, my advice is to only start deeper, more direct cranial techniques when the patient has had quite a few treatments and the practitioner feels that they will be able to cope.

Other manual techniques

This chapter has touched upon the osteopathic techniques that I use in the treatment of long COVID. There are a few other manual techniques that I sometimes employ when necessary, depending on the individual case. One such technique is abdominal massage.

Many long COVID patients complain of irritable bowel syndrome, therefore, if the patient is suffering from severe bowel symptoms, such as pain and bloating, or the surface abdominal lymphatic vessels feel congested and varicose, then I may use the following mild abdominal massage technique: using plenty of lubricating oil or cream, I will gently massage the tummy following the pathway of the large intestine, first going up on the right side of the patient then across the top of the abdomen to the left and then down. This slow clockwise motion is repeated for a minute or two and then, to avoid any stagnation in the inguinal lymph nodes, immediately followed by effleurage from both sides of the lower abdomen up over the chest to the central drainage just under the clavicles.

In the past I have had some patients write to me about all sorts of treatments that they couldn't find in my books and were wondering if this was a good idea. It may be that further down the line, as the patient progresses, an experienced practitioner may wish to add other manual techniques of their own to the sessions with the patient. There may possibly be techniques specific to the patient's requirements or some procedures that have helped others. As long as they promote improved drainage of the lymphatics as well as blood flow and do not encourage any backflow of the central lymph they can be gradually added to the Perrin Technique™ protocol, but with extreme caution, to avoid too quick a detoxification or overloading the sympathetic nervous system by too vigorous a technique.

It is important for the practitioner to explain to the patient which extra techniques not mentioned in this book are being done and form no part of the Perrin Technique™.

After treatment

Immediately after standard treatment the patient may feel slightly giddy and possibly even nauseous. To avoid fainting or being too disorientated they should first lie on their side, gently swing their legs over the edge of the treatment table and slowly sit up from the side-lying position. They should then have a slight rest just sitting at the side of the treatment table with their feet on the floor for a minimum of 10 seconds before trying to get up from the treatment plinth. Some long COVID patients may need to rest for about a minute or longer before standing up following a treatment session as they suffer from 'orthostatic intolerance' which refers to a group of clinical conditions due to sympathetic nerve disturbance in which symptoms worsen with upright posture and are reduced when lying down. The severe form of orthostatic intolerance is known as 'postural orthostatic tachycardia syndrome' (POTS) and is discussed on pages 57–59.

Some patients need a drink of water to help their nausea and dizziness directly after the session. This is due to the fact that this treatment 'does what it says on the tin'. Real poisons/toxins are being released from the central nervous system during the half hour or so of the treatment session. The body has to be able to cope and we help the detox programme with a few choice supplements that should relieve many of the nasty side effects of this process. As the French artist Paul Cézanne and the animated character Shrek famously said, 'Better out than in'. However, another adage, 'Less is more', originally from a poem by Robert Browning and made famous by architect Ludwig Miles van der Rohe, encompasses one of my golden rules for treatment long COVID.

IMPORTANT NOTE TO PRACTITIONERS When doing the Perrin Technique™, always apply the rule of 'LESS IS MORE', especially concerning cranio-sacral treatment. Particularly in the early stages of treatment, care should be taken not to over-stimulate the drainage, especially the cranial rhythm, with too long or forceful a treatment as one might drain off excess toxins at one session, causing too much of a severe reaction. As the therapeutic programme progresses and the patient improves, the practitioner can gradually increase the intensity of treatment and, if necessary, use additional techniques.

Conclusion

The Perrin Technique™, in a nutshell, has been developed to help drain the inflammatory toxins away from the central nervous system and incorporates gentle manual techniques that stimulate the healthy flow of lymphatic and cerebrospinal fluid and improve spinal mechanics. This in turn reduces the toxic overload to the brain which subsequently reduces the strain on the sympathetic nervous system, and this ultimately supports a return to good health.[27, 28, 29, 30]

Supplementing treatment with self-help

As explained above, manual treatment improves the function of the thorax and the spine and thereby the functioning of lymphatic drainage. This is especially so when enhanced by routine mobility exercises that the patient regularly undertakes. Some effective exercises to improve and maintain the quality of movement of the dorsal spine areas are described in Chapter 7 which is addressed to patients in plain English, and also shown on the new online video, freely available online (see page 205 for further details). These are very important as they will encourage better drainage down the spine and out through the perivascular spaces in the blood vessels supplying each spinal nerve. These simple exercises should be continued even when all the symptoms have abated and you need no further treatment.

Chapter 5

The recovery process

'Navigation was always a difficult art,
Though with only one ship and one bell:
And he feared he must really decline, for his part,
Undertaking another as well.'

Lewis Carroll

The Hunting of The Snark

Case: Antonia's story

In early 2020, amidst the onset of the pandemic, I experienced a range of symptoms (including breathing issues and severe gland pain) following exposure to COVID-19. Initially misdiagnosed as panic attacks, my symptoms persisted for months, evolving into suspected viral complications including nerve pain and a rash. Despite repeated hospital visits, my concerns were dismissed until I developed worsened heart palpitations, food intolerances and a series of severe kidney infections. Eventually I was diagnosed with mast cell activation syndrome, EDS and POTS that were exacerbated by COVID-19, and from which I continued to struggle with chronic pain and fatigue.

In June 2022, I sought treatment from osteopath, Kosta Kolimechkov, who introduced me to the Perrin Technique™. Having endured glandular fever and ME in my early 20s, my health had never fully recovered.

My initial Perrin-Juhl ME/CFS score was 3/10 with a score of 223 when answering 'the profile of fatigue-related states (PFRS)' which reflected the profound health issues I was experiencing, and by August 2023 it had improved to 111 (and 5/10 respectively) and now it is at 58.

The Perrin Technique™ has finally brought the relief that I haven't found elsewhere. My nerve pain has diminished, the kidney and bladder pain has improved and my energy has returned. Weekly treatments and self-massage techniques taught by Kosta, along with studying Dr Perrin's books provided a path to recovery.

For the first time, I felt understood and supported by a practitioner. Through Kosta's expertise and compassion and artful application of the Perrin Technique™, I've regained hope for a healthy, functional body after years of feeling dismissed and misunderstood. I am so grateful to feel more in control of my body than ever before.

Antonia Peck, Richmond, London, UK.
Patient of Licensed Perrin Technique™ practitioner Kosta Kolimechkov

Getting worse before getting better

One proof that the Perrin Technique™ is not a placebo is the fact that most patients feel a great deal worse at the beginning of their treatment. Placebo treatments generally do not make you feel worse. The reason for this initial exacerbation in the symptoms is that, as well as draining out the pro-inflammatory cytokines that built up during a COVID-19 infection, other large molecular toxins embedded (possibly for years) in the central nervous system are being released into the rest of the body. As mentioned earlier, we need the lymphatic system and the glymphatic system to drain away macro-molecules such as cytokines, which are large protein molecules.

Headaches and pain can occur. This is because the treatment encourages the toxins to leave the brain, they will initially affect the superficial tissues in the head and, as they drain down to the rest of the body, pain may follow. We know from the earlier studies of the glymphatic system by the research team at Rochester University in New York, that the first points of toxic build-up when the drainage stops are the thalamus and the basal ganglia, which are the gateway of sensory input and control of pain perception from around the body. So, any pain felt by the patient due to stimulation of any nociceptor (pain receptor) outside the brain is exaggerated.

Another unpleasant sign that occurs when the body's drainage is improving is the appearance of spots, boils and other skin eruptions. Until the lymphatic channels are working properly, the toxins have to go somewhere and the quickest way out of the body is often through the skin. These normally clear up as the treatment progresses. Some patients in the past have suffered from severe acne which occurs when the oil from sebaceous glands blocks hair follicles in the skin. Bacteria which infect the plugged follicles, causing the pustules seen in acne, may resurface with treatment and re-infect the hair follicles leading to a resurgence of the acne.

The first few weeks, or sometimes months in severe cases, are always the most trying for the patient. In clinic I have often noticed that the worse the patient is in the early stages of treatment, the better, usually, it bodes for their prognosis as the toxins flow out of the central nervous system. However, we need the patient to cope with the side effects and, if the reaction is too unpleasant and the patient suffers too much, it can be counterproductive.

The Perrin Technique™ is patient-centred at all times. It is important that the practitioner listens to the patient and initially goes very softly with the treatment. If the patient is in too much pain with the initial treatment, or other symptoms become unbearable, the practitioner should lessen the treatment intensity and sometimes space out the treatment sessions to a level where the patient can cope.

Paradoxically, some patients respond better when the treatment is more intense and more frequent. As I have stated frequently in this book, every long COVID patient is different. Both patient and practitioner can work out the routine that suits the patient's condition and achieve the best results in the longer term.

The main aspects for long COVID sufferers to focus upon are the changes occurring during the treatment. (If change has not occurred in any way during the first 12 weeks of treatment, the patient may have to take an alternative route in their search for a cure.) My treatment often hugely improves the patient's health, but most will need other treatments in tandem in order to alleviate all symptoms. I have noticed that other treatments – whether they be based on nutrition or pharmaceuticals – work better after the patient's neuro-lymphatic pathways have improved. Patients who have tried supplements before treatment, to no avail, are advised to try some of the supplements again after undergoing the Perrin Technique™, as they may now prove more effective.

The jigsaw puzzle analogy

As no two long COVID patients are ever the same, there are many different approaches that can be helpful when used in conjunction with my treatment. The analogy I like to use to explain the importance of treating the neuro-lymphatic dysfunction in long COVID is that of a jigsaw puzzle (see Fig. 23).

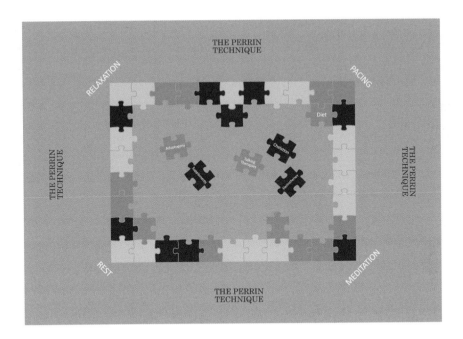

Fig. 23 The jigsaw puzzle analogy (see also Plate 4).

When one tries to complete a jigsaw puzzle, it is best to start with the corners and edge pieces first. The four corners of the recovery jigsaw puzzle in long COVID are:

- rest
- relaxation
- meditation/mindfulness
- pacing.

Rest

During the day patients should spend some time, preferably at least three times a day, in complete rest, in a darkened room if possible, with no sound and taking time out from everything. This could be for a few minutes or longer if the patient needs more time to switch off.

It is no good if patients lie down and rest thinking 'I'm resting …yes, I'm resting because that's what Dr Perrin says you have to do! … yes, I'm resting RESTING… RESTING…RESTING!!!!'

Relax

You have to relax when resting. The best word for it is chillax just like these fortunate Swedes who I saw on one of my lecture trips and who have definitely worked out how to destress and chillax with the aid of these Stockholm children (see Fig. 24).

Meditation

If you cannot relax due to many stress factors in your life, then use meditation techniques such as mindfulness. Follow the advice of Confucius who famously said, 'The past is history, the future's a mystery, the present a gift'. Focus on the here and now and something that is good.

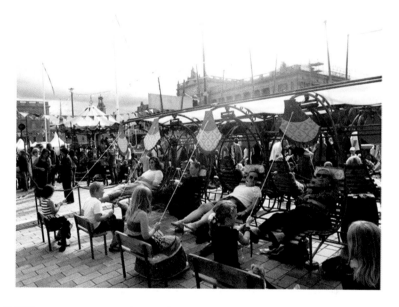

Fig. 24 These parents and grandparents in Stockholm know the meaning of 'chillax' with these rocking chairs and fans controlled by the children!

Mindfulness is a therapeutic meditation technique that improves mental wellbeing by focusing on the present moment as well as calmly acknowledging and accepting one's feelings, thoughts and bodily sensations plus awareness of the world around one.

There are plenty of books and online audio and video self-help guides to mindfulness. One of the books I was recommended by a colleague was *Dancing With Elephants* by Jarem Sawatsky[1] which is full of excellent advice and help in mindfulness training for anyone with a chronic illness.

Near the end of the book the author talks about another author of self-help books, Toni Bernhard, a past law professor in California who was chronically ill for many years and used mindfulness to help her, saying that we always need to be kind to ourselves and are often too quick to lose our temper with ourselves. How often do people call themselves stupid or feel terribly cross with themselves if they make a silly mistake? They are often more angry than if another family member or friend made the same error, but this is the nature of many long COVID patients who are often feeling guilty about being ill and not being a help to those closest to them.

Many patients with long COVID are similar to ME/CFS patients, in suffering from TPOS (thoroughly p****d off syndrome) which is a name that, although it usually brings a smile to my patients' faces, resonates with them as they often feel helpless and frustrated beyond belief; they want to, but cannot, get on with their lives as any attempt to try and beat the disease is hit by a brick wall … a very large and impassable brick wall. This is not helped by blaming oneself for having the illness.

The main take away from Sawatsky's marvellous tome is that patients with long-term problems such as long COVID should start by loving themselves and practise more self-compassion. So, start loving yourself and focus on anything positive, concentrating on the here and now. This is not a cure by itself but a major component in improving the health of long COVID sufferers.

Even if you can't relax, using meditation can often enhance your chillax session. There are many meditative techniques and mindfulness programs that you can try out online if you can't get to a live class to learn the skills needed to get the best out of meditation.

There is much evidence to suggest meditative states are effective and sustainable in reducing fatigue, unrefreshing sleep and inflammation, whilst also enhancing immunity in post-viral fatigue, including long COVID.[2]

Pacing

In 1989, when doctors were generally telling ME/CFS patients to exercise more, I advised patients to pace. Since then, I have been banging on from every conference centre rooftop for three decades that ME/CFS patients should pace, and not follow the old guideline of graded exercise (GET), which has finally been dropped by the NHS in the UK. Pacing means doing half of all physical and mental activities that you think you can do (the '50%' or 'half rule') as mentioned previously. The same 50% rule follows with long COVID.

Pacing, by the way, does not mean, as one doctor I met at a conference thought, 'pacing up and down in a corridor'.

I swam against the tide in 1989 by advising patients with ME/CFS to pace and reduce their activity, an approach which I have championed ever since. However, significant improvement has been shown when patients are advised to avoid too much activity and carry out only 50% of their perceived capabilities. In the early 1990s, when most of the medical fraternity believed ME/CFS was just lack of general fitness or a form of depression and were therefore advocating exercise for ME/CFS, when patients who could hardly walk were advised to get fitter, I was instructing all ME/CFS sufferers to stop and pace themselves, doing just half of whatever they felt they were capable of, whether it was walking, talking or watching TV.

My 'half rule' remains a major influence on the long COVID patient's overall improvement with my treatment. If the patient overdoes things during the course of treatment, they may never fully recover; indeed, their health may worsen. Some patients tell me they find it difficult to gauge what half is. Often, they have realised that they are doing too much after the particular activity and it is too late. One patient who was a keen swimmer was given the go-ahead to go back into the pool as part of her reconditioning programme and instead of keeping to the half rule, she swam 50 lengths on her first dip. Her symptoms raised their ugly head again, and it took her weeks to recover. I asked her did she think she could have done 100 lengths? She admitted that she couldn't have managed 60, so she should have swum a maximum of 25 – that is, half of what she felt capable of doing – and even then, I would have suggested starting with just a few lengths.

The best way of following the 'half rule' is by thinking double. If you walk 0.5 km, ask yourself, 'Can I honestly walk 1 km with no problem?' If the answer is no, 0.5 km is too much. If 1 km receives an emphatic 'yes' with no worsening of the symptoms, 0.5 km is fine. If you are uncertain, even 0.5 km may be too much, you should reduce the distance. The same applies to any activity – for example, having a conversation: if half an hour is too much, engage in only 10-minute chats at any one time. If a two-hour film is too long, use the device you are watching it on to view half-hour sections at a time, provided that you feel you could watch an hour without adverse effects. This strategy prevents you from overstressing your sympathetic nervous system and, although it is difficult to implement, I have found this to be the golden rule that may make the difference between just helping a person a little, to actually getting them back to good health. As the patient improves, then they can gradually increase activity safely as long as they stick by the 'half rule' … as I constantly tell my patients 'half of more is still more!'

The edge pieces of the jigsaw puzzle

The edge pieces of the puzzle are the treatment protocol that is the Perrin Technique™, described in Chapters 4 and 7, correcting the biomechanics and improving the neuro-lymphatic drainage and thus creating a framework for the rest of the picture to be filled in by the internal pieces which represent all the supplements, medications and talk therapies plus other treatment that may help (see Chapters 8 and 9).

Sometimes the jigsaw puzzle of recovery is made up of only corners and edges, or just a few pieces in the middle, which makes the task much more straightforward and represents a patient making a complete recovery with just my standard advice and treatment.

Unfortunately, most cases are much more complex, with many difficult sections to be filled in. The supplements, medications, diets and talk therapies all form part of the internal pieces in the jigsaw puzzle picture of health.

One can of course start with the centre of a challenging puzzle first, but it will make the task much more difficult, and one might give up before the picture is complete. Sometimes it seems too difficult and there are so many symptoms and problems that the practitioner doesn't know where to begin. So, start with the corners and edges to bring about the best result.

Frequency of treatment

At the beginning of treatment, it is important that the patient is treated once a week and that the treatment remains regular and weekly, together with all the home massage and other self-help routines described in detail in Chapter 7. This usually carries on for at least the first 12 weeks and, slowly, as the symptom picture improves, there is a gradual increase in the time between consultations. With very severe cases, weekly treatments may be necessary for much longer than three months. Eventually, when patients remain symptom-free between their six-monthly check-ups and are able to perform all reasonable activities, doing all they could do before they were ill with no side effects, I will score them 10 out of 10 using the scale described below. This is difficult to achieve, but it does happen every so often and is a wonderful feeling for both sufferer and practitioner. When I discharge the 10/10 patients it gives me the motivation and strength to carry on my clinical work treating some very severe bed-ridden patients and continue my research into ME/CFS, FMS and long COVID.

While acknowledging that every patient is different, the chart described below (see Table 5.1, page 142), which is based on the general severity of the illness, is a guide that both the patient and practitioner can use when calculating the overall prognosis.

Table 5.1 is a sliding scale and should be used as a general guide. In other words, if a patient initially scores 5/10 on long COVID alone, and is also suffering from another disorder, the overall score may be 4/10 or lower. If the physical findings during the examination are very evident and apparent, the overall score is lowered. As I have said, I often find that the patient is trying to appear healthier than they really are. This fits the profile of the average long COVID sufferer who tries as hard as they can to keep going until, eventually, they have to admit they cannot go on any further or they will just collapse.

In 2014, Dr John Juhl, DO, an osteopathic physician in New York, who attended my workshop on the Perrin Technique™, posed the following challenge. He argued that the score 0–10 should accurately correlate with the patient's history and overall condition rather than just rely on a score based on my experience and should also focus mainly on the patient's quality of life.

I agreed wholeheartedly with him. He said, 'It seems important both to give the patient a sense of whether they have the diagnosis at their initial office visit, and how long they should expect the treatment to last.' This is important and I could see it being difficult for a practitioner new to my Technique to make an accurate score that was reliable.

So, in 2014, I set to work for a few months analysing dozens of initial scores that I had given in prior cases. I devised a weighted scoring system that I adapted to reflect the different factors that led me to a reasonably accurate initial score for most patients; I further updated this in 2019. This new four-part scoring system delivers an objective method of determining a more precise overall prognosis that can be used by all trained practitioners. Although developed for ME/CFS, this scoring system can be adapted for long COVID.

The Perrin-Juhl scoring system

A. Long COVID symptoms

The first score we calculate is the number of common symptoms of long COVID that a patient has. This is achieved by using the general health questionnaire devised for my initial clinical trial, the 50-symptom Perrin Questionnaire for chronic fatigue syndrome/ME (PQ-CFS).[3]

Note that the PQ-CFS maximum scores are:

- Adult female = 49
- Adult male = 47 (as no symptoms would be reported related to menses).

The maximum scores are not 50 and 48 since long COVID does not cause joint swelling (question 16 on the questionnaire), so patients with only long COVID will not place a tick for this symptom. If they do, it means that there is a comorbidity (another condition) that is some form of arthritic condition, and thus they would add the score for that comorbidity to the PQ-CFS score – see part B.

B. Comorbidities

The next part of the Perrin-Juhl scoring system reflects the impact of other conditions that may be present together with long COVID.

For **each** comorbidity add the following to the PQ-CFS score in part A:

- if minor impact + 5
- if moderate impact + 10
- if severely affected + 20.

C. Quality of life

One should then analyse how the patient's life has been affected by their various symptoms/comorbidities and factor that into the overall calculation, as follows.

Add the following to the total scores from Part A and Part B:

- Able to continue as normal + 0
- Only able to work part-time/struggling to cope with work + 5
- Unable to work but not housebound + 10
- Housebound + 20
- Totally bedridden + 40.

D. Longevity of symptoms

Add the following score to reflect the time the patient has suffered from their symptom(s):

- Under 12 months + 0
- 1–5 years + 5
- 5–10 years + 10
- More than 10 years + 20.

Obviously, at the time of writing this book in 2024, nobody will have suffered from long COVID for more than four years, but as time goes on patients without the appropriate treatment may worsen with time and in a few years may score + 10 or + 20.

Calculate a total score by working through parts A–D, then convert this to a score out of 10 using Table 5.1.

Table 5.1 Conversion chart

Total score	Severity of long COVID
125+	1/10
101–124	1.5/10
81–100	2/10
71–80	2.5/10
61–70	3/10
51–60	3.5/10
46–50	4/10
41–45	4.5/10
36–40	5/10
31–35	5.5/10
26–30	6/10
21–25	6.5/10
16–20	7/10

As patients show a significant change in their symptoms or their quality of life improves, then it will change the scores. Equally, if they recover from their comorbidity then the long COVID score will improve.

I, and other practitioners, can expect to see very few new patients over 7/10 as they are just about coping and usually do not see the reason to seek medical help.

Later on in the treatment, as the patient improves, a score above 7 represents the patient's ability to do more normal things without experiencing worsening symptoms, which is reflected in Table 5.2 on the overall prognosis for the illness.

Also, most important: if using the new Perrin-Juhl scoring system, and you find the patient hasn't scored too high (e.g. 39) but is clearly suffering more severely than the converted 5/10 score suggests, then a physical examination usually helps to produce a more accurate score. For example, if the physical signs are very noticeable and palpable, then the long COVID severity score should be reduced by 1, so in this example the patient would score a 4/10 rather than 5/10 which should give a more accurate prognosis, as shown in Table 5.2.

Table 5.2 The outlook

Score	Description	Prognosis
1	Extreme symptoms and signs for more than a year. Totally bedridden or sitting all day, little cranial flow palpable.	3 years +
2	Severe symptoms and signs for more than a year. Bedridden or sitting all day, little cranial flow palpable.	2 years+
3	Severe symptoms and signs for more than a year, resting most of the day, little cranial flow palpable.	2 years
4	Severe symptoms and signs for 6–12 months, resting most of the day, little cranial flow palpable.	18 months+
5	Severe symptoms and signs for at least 3 months; able to carry out light tasks but requires regular rest periods.	12–18 months
6	Moderate symptoms and signs for at least 3 months; able to work part-time with a struggle.	8–12 months
7	Moderate symptoms and signs for at least 3 months; able to work full-time with difficulty.	8 months
8	Moderate symptoms and signs for at least 3 months; daily life slightly limited. Symptoms worsen on activity.	6 months
9	No symptoms but still signs of slight lymphatic engorgement and experiences mild symptoms following over-exertion.	3 months
10	Symptom-free for at least 6 months. Able to live a full active life ... within reason.	Discharged

Conclusion

As we can see, there is no 'one cap fits all' or 'magic bullet' approach to beating long COVID, as every individual patient has a unique set of symptoms due to the individuality of the condition, with myriads of different toxins affecting trillions of combinations of neurological pathways in the brain. The Perrin Technique™ offers a treatment and self-help programme that helps most, but isn't a cure-all approach. It involves a patient-practitioner partnership, where the treatment is always patient-centred but often takes time to show its benefit. Most patients with long COVID are helped by the Perrin Technique™ and some in a matter of weeks or months. However, this condition is a chronic illness and can take years and a multidisciplinary approach to achieve the desired result.

In February 2024, George Lundberg MD wrote a very apt article on long COVID calling it, 'Another Great Pretender',[4] stating that the medical profession as a whole do not really understand this disease. He asked in his commentary: 'Did you or do you now have long COVID? How do you know? Do you even know what long COVID is? How would you diagnose?'

Hopefully Dr Lundberg and other doctors trying to piece all the symptomatic jigsaw puzzle pieces together will finally realise that long COVID is a disease affecting the neuro-lymphatic system. As shown in this book, stimulating a healthy lymphatic drainage of the brain and spinal cord is paramount in helping these patients, leading to symptomatic relief and a better quality of life, with some achieving full recovery from this misunderstood disease.

Chapter 6

Can long COVID be cured?

'Down, down, down. Would the fall never come to an end!'

Lewis Carrol

Alice's Adventures in Wonderland

Case: Kat's story

I got first got COVID in June 2021. I had the typical flu-like symptoms of feeling hot, achy, with a sore throat and lethargy. After two weeks of being able to do very little other than rest in bed, I began to feel less acute and hoped that this was the beginning of my recovery. However, very little changed. I was beginning to panic as the symptoms swiftly developed into signs of long COVID – intense fatigue, brain fog, aches, speech issues, tinnitus, digestive problems, appetite disappearance, the works.

Before catching Covid I had been a very healthy and active 40-year-old. My work as an actor was very intense and required high energy as well as a good memory to remember lines. None of that had been a problem. I used to go the gym and generally my life was high energy. However, now I was feeling completely zapped of all energy. I had incredible brain fog. I couldn't even string sentences together. My energy was non-existent. Even doing the most sedentary things was making me feel like I had climbed a mountain.

As the weeks progressed I became very stressed with what seemed like a never-ending situation. Nothing was improving. I could barely look after myself and was struggling to even prepare food. I was convinced by my parents to move back home where I could be looked after and nursed back to health. Even with all this extra care, nothing was helping and I had to give up work as I just was incapable of the journey let alone doing anything.

I tried a few things, some of which helped; changing my diet impacted me a lot. It was a very scary time. As I've described, I went from being a very healthy, very fit, non-stop very active person to being someone that could barely walk for more than a few minutes and had to have their meals cooked for them.

In my few moments of limited mental and physical energy I began to do some research and look for anything that could help me out of this really dreadful existence.

I am forever profoundly grateful that I found the wonderful Sophie King. Nothing has helped me move forward more than her expertise with the Perrin Technique™ and her understanding of long COVID. She explained in a lot of detail how the COVID virus had damaged the healthy flow in my lymphatic system and that my body was in a constantly toxic state. I visited Sophie for weekly appointments and religiously did all my self-massage routine at home. I have improved incredibly. I can now work a little, and travel on trains without then crashing, I can go to the gym a few times a week, I can speak with friends for more than an hour! I know these achievements sound small to someone who lives a 'normal' life, but these are huge, huge improvements from not being able to do literally anything all day. I would encourage anyone with long COVID to try the Perrin Technique™ and get back on the road to health.

Katharine Bennett, Dorset, UK.
Patient of Licensed Perrin Technique™ practitioner, Sophie King

The magic bullet?

Will there ever be one pill to cure long COVID? This question is raised again and again by patients, doctors and scientists. In my opinion, based on over 35 years of clinical research into the field of ME/CFS, the answer is unfortunately but unequivocally, NO! This is because every long COVID patient is different, with the inflammatory cytokines affecting different neurochemical pathways, in turn affecting different sections of the central nervous system, causing different metabolic disturbances, leading to a different array of symptoms. This view, as you can imagine, makes me hugely popular at scientific meetings and conferences … Not!

Of course, nobody wants to hear this, or read this for that matter, and for the patient it looks as if all is lost.

But it isn't!

It just means that we have to approach the treatment of long COVID in a different way to most diseases. As leading Canadian ME/CFS physician, the late Dr Bruce Carruthers, once said regarding ME/CFS, 'Treat the dis-ease and not the disease!'

'Big Pharma', a colloquial term for leading pharmaceutical firms that produce most of our medicines today, don't like to hear this either. If there is not a potential huge return on investment, they may not be motivated to help research the disease and potential treatments in the first place. If there is little chance of a magic bullet to kill the bug or sort out the biochemical problem, then they won't see the point of funding studies that go on for many years before any successful pill or potion may be developed. One can hardly blame them – they are commercial organisations.

There are, however, blood and other lab tests and drugs that have been and are being developed that will identify and help some sub-groups of patients, such as targeting an aspect of the immune system or reducing the upregulated stress response. These may help some patients, but unfortunately worsen other individuals with long COVID who have a different symptom picture with other metabolic disturbances.

As explained in Chapter 2, there are two major and complex problems that continue to beset the diagnosis and treatment of long COVID:

- The first is that two or more conditions can co-exist at any one time in one patient. It is sometimes difficult for doctors to distinguish between, for example, depression and long COVID, particularly in those cases of long COVID in which depression is an additional feature.
- The second problem is that, because there is no universally accepted means of diagnosis by tests such as blood or urine analysis, most doctors diagnose long COVID based on a history of a past infection by COVID-19 and, when all other possible diagnoses have been excluded. In my view, this is a hazardous method of diagnosing any disease. Can you imagine if a doctor were to tell a patient, 'Well, after all the tests, we cannot find anything else wrong with you, so it must be cancer.' Yet millions of people around the world are being told that they have long COVID using the exclusion method of diagnosis.

Conversely, many others are being diagnosed as having long COVID far too quickly due to the fact the symptoms began after the infection of COVID-19 without testing whether the patient actually has any other possible pathology. Both these approaches could lead to patients receiving the wrong diagnosis and, worst of all, inappropriate treatment that may endanger them.

Some medical experts on long COVID have touched upon the neurological effects of the disease, and how the immune system and the body's hormones are affected. However, the treatment recommended by these specialists is to improve the immune system by pharmacological methods or affect chemical balance by dietary means, supplements or, if necessary, by psychiatric drugs or psychotherapy. These treatments do help symptom relief in many cases and often I will recommend supplementation and agree with many pharmaceutical approaches to help certain symptoms, but if this is all that is done to treat the patient, then these practitioners are missing a crucial point: they are treating just the body's long-term response to the infection, i.e. the symptoms rather than aiming at the root cause of the disorder. The neurological system that controls the chemical balance of the body is the autonomic nervous system and the system that is the main factor in drainage of major toxins from the body as well as a major part of our immune system is the lymphatic system. If these two systems were working correctly, the body would cope better with extra stresses and strains due to chemical, physical, mental, immunological and emotional exertion. Only then might pharmacological approaches, such as anti-inflammatories or immunotherapy, psychotherapy or healthy hypoallergenic diets, bring about a permanent improvement in patients with long COVID.

Sadly, in many people with this condition, there is little or no recovery, despite many and varied dietary and chemical approaches to treatment. The key to finding a complete and lasting remedy is to find a treatment that helps the body cope with the extra load. This concept is in keeping with modern medicine's approach to the management of COVID-19 itself and other types of disease: for example, the use of vaccinations to increase the body's immunity, and thus resist the effects of many infections such as COVID-19, especially when the body is attacked by a high viral load of the SARS-CoV-2 coronavirus.

The SLYM

Although I have discovered a way of helping patients with long COVID, the sad fact is that in most cases the drainage of toxins in the central nervous system via the Perrin Technique™ takes a long time, and unfortunately, in the majority of patients, the central nervous system cannot be fully cleansed. Why is this? Why can't I just do the treatment to help drainage of the brain, remove the toxins and, hey presto, within a few days or weeks the patient is completely cured?

My initial answer was that in some patients there are many deeply engrained toxins in the brain, and it takes a long time to remove the toxic soup made up of possibly thousands of harmful chemicals that have either been overproduced within the patient or invaded the body and may yet still be entering the unfortunate patient.

However, this answer has never sat easily with me as some patients have followed all my advice and had many detox treatments on top of the Perrin Technique™ and still, after years, have many symptoms that need regular treatment.

This very perplexing question has been a source of angst over the years and was only finally explained at the beginning of 2023.

A new part of the brain's neuro-lymphatic system has been discovered by scientists at the University of Copenhagen in Denmark.[1] This is a thin layer of tissue lying above the pia called the subarachnoid lymphatic-like membrane, or SLYM, which was mentioned in Chapter 2. This separates fresh cerebrospinal fluid from fluid containing waste products.

It is an extremely thin layer, just a few cells wide or, in places, just one cell, and is loaded with immune cells to enable it to be an early defence against infection in the cerebrospinal fluid. This subarachnoid space is not only in the brain, but also forms a major part of the membrane of the spinal cord, ending at the second sacral segment at the base of the spine.

So, what I believe is happening with many long COVID patients is that, in the past, they have had trauma (possibly repetitive) or long-term inflammation (possibly due to infection) that has irreparably damaged the SLYM in the cranium or the spine.

Physical trauma to this thin layer of tissue, even perhaps at birth, could affect the integrity of the CSF and pollute the healthy CSF with inflammatory toxins, which could explain prolonged neuro-inflammation and the increased risk of developing neuro-lymphatic disorders following earlier physical trauma to the head and spine. Then, when applying my techniques, some toxins drain away out of the central nervous system, but some will pass back into the brain through the injured SLYM.

My theory could explain why some people suffer badly from effects of a lumbar puncture (spinal tap) where the doctor will push a needle into the subarachnoid space in the spine to extract cerebrospinal fluid. Until last year nobody knew about the existence of the SLYM so the needle in most cases would pierce this delicate membrane, potentially leading to major health problems in the future and susceptibility to neuro-lymphatic diseases such as long COVID (see Fig. 25).

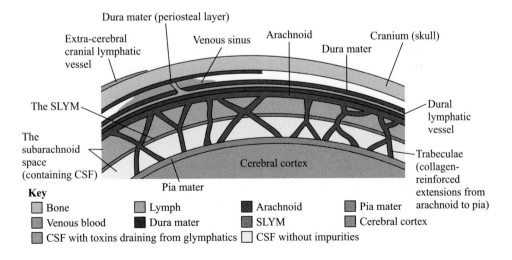

Fig. 25 Cross-section of the skull (top) and outer layer of the brain, showing the subarachnoid lymphatic-like membrane (SLYM).[1] (See also Plate 5.)

If there is a backflow of lymph in long COVID, beside the varicose megalymphatics felt in the chest of patients, we should also see enlarged perivascular spaces in the brain of these patients. Sure enough, the first paper to demonstrate radiological evidence of brain changes in long COVID,[2] showed unequivocally that there were enlarged perivascular spaces in the basal ganglia – an area in the mid brain that was shown to be affected 10 years before when the glymphatic system was stopped from working (see Fig. 26).[3]

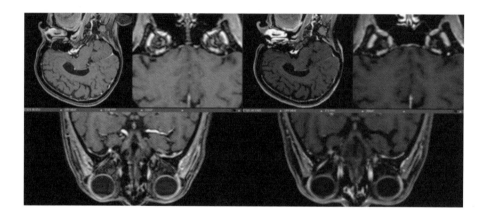

Fig. 26 Enlarged perivascular spaces. Prominent perivascular spaces in the right greater than left basal ganglia were visualised on MRI.[2]

Another important recent discovery is that the brainstem volume has been shown to be increased in long COVID, which researchers have possibly linked to oedema, due to inflammatory changes.[4] Obviously, if there is a backflow in the lymphatic system, the swollen perivascular spaces will produce a visibly larger volume in the brain. Lymphoedema is most commonly found in the lower part of the legs due to gravitational effects, so it is possible that gravity could play an important part in the cerebrospinal fluid build-up within the brainstem and can be further aggravated by a build-up of intra-cranial pressure.[5]

The CSF canalicular system

Another major discovery published in 2023 regarding the drainage of cerebrospinal fluid has further validated my management and treatment of long COVID. The original model of cerebrospinal fluid (CSF) drainage in humans was that it drains from the subarachnoid space into the sagittal sinus vein. Then in 2017 the lymphatic system of the human brain was proven and so we then had two pathways of CSF drainage.

Dr Joel Pessa, a retired plastic surgeon from Texas, noticed during his many years of operating on the head and neck of patents, two visible canals running through the tissue of the neck lying alongside the internal jugular veins. In recent years he has been looking at what these canals are. The craziest thing about this discovery is that these canals can be seen with the naked eye and, unbelievably with all the thousands of anatomists and surgeons over the years, nobody bothered before to find out what these canals were. Together with an anatomist, Dr Pessa injected fluid into the canals of cadavers showing that they contain cerebrospinal fluid and drain the CSF with the aid of gravity from the subarachnoid space down to the subclavian veins.[6]

Interestingly, Dr Pessa has also published research using nanoprobes that has followed the flow of cerebrospinal fluid along epineural channels adjacent to peripheral nerves all over the body draining into subcutaneous lymphatic vessels lying alongside small superficial nerves.[7] The clinical implications of these findings could lead to understanding more about peripheral neuropathy which affects some long COVID patients on top of sympathetic-induced nerve irritation via ephapses already discussed in Chapter 4.[8]

And talking of gravity, a conversation I had recently at a dinner party somehow got onto the subject of the moon's gravitational effect on tides, especially during the full moon. So, I wondered could the lunar gravitational pull increase the backflow of fluid into the brain's lymphatic drainage?

The derogatory term 'lunatic' was commonly used from the 16th to the 18th centuries in England for people whose mental health seemed to be affected cyclically and was thought to be caused by the moon. The term comes from the Latin 'luna'. But, as absurd as it sounds, maybe the moons gravitational pull can affect the CSF in the minute passages of this canalicular system and the glymphatic drainage system (see Fig. 27).

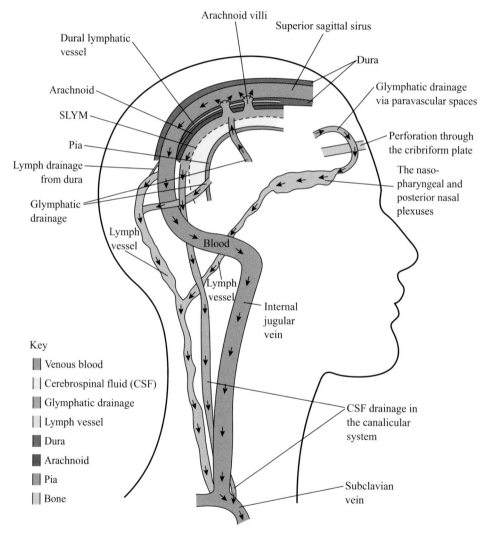

Fig. 27 A schematic diagram showing the key drainage pathways from the brain. (See also Plate 6.)

The lunar effects could increase the congestion and backflow, especially when this system is already disturbed as in long COVID. It would be very interesting to know how many patients do feel worse when there is a full moon.

So, Dr Pessa's discovery of the canalicular system running down the neck will explain why patients who are very severely ill and lying down flat all day are actually harming themselves further. If severe patients were able to sit up even for a short while, then the canalicular system would be able to help drain away some toxins via CSF just by gravity.

I recently attended a major conference in the USA where other long COVID experts were discussing how severe patients are monitored regarding possible improvement. Some use an index related to how long in a day the patient sits up in bed as opposed to lying flat. As the patient improved, the amount of time sitting up increased. I explained to my fellow scientists that the amount of time sitting up was not only a measurement of improvement but the probable reason for the actual improvement by aiding the drainage of the canalicular system and reducing the amount of inflammatory toxins in the brain.

Dr Pessa's discovery also underpins why the effleurage down the neck plays such an important role in the Perrin Technique™ as it not only helps the brain drain toxins through the lymphatics, but it also manually helps the drainage down the CSF canalicular system, especially for those very severe patients who cannot even lift their heads off a pillow.

Potential role of nitric oxide

Recently a scientific discovery in South Korea has shown in glorious technicolour the exact route and mechanism in the brain that underpins my original theory of the sympathetic nervous system dysfunction causing a disturbed neuro-lymphatic flow in ME/CFS. A crucial network of lymphatic vessels at the back of the nose, known as the nasopharyngeal and posterior nasal lymphatic plexuses, have been shown to be the major drainage pathway of cerebrospinal fluid (CSF) from the brain into the deeper cervical lymphatics.

This ground-breaking study led by Dr Gou Young Koh, director of the Center for Vascular Research at South Korean's Institute for Basic Science, used cutting-edge science on the brains of mice, imaging the intricate network of lymphatic vessels which then drain large amounts of cerebrospinal fluid into the cervical lymph vessels which are controlled by the sympathetic nervous system.[9] A similar study came out nearly the same week led by Dr Steven T Proulx at the University of Bern in Switzerland (see Fig 27).[10]

The researchers in Korea showed that increasing nitric oxide or a dose of medication that stimulates noradrenaline/norepinephrine aids sympathetic control of the cervical lymphatic vessels that drain from the nasopharyngeal lymphatic plexus. This, the authors claim, indicates the possible use of drugs to help increase sympathetic tone for neurodegenerative disorders such as Alzheimer's. However, as with long COVID, it is not a sluggish lymphatic system that leads to these neurodegenerative or neuro-immune diseases, but, as shown in this book, it is a reversal of lymphatic drainage by a dysfunctional neurological control that is at the root of these disorders. Drugs to stimulate this flow could cause more drainage in the wrong direction, leading to further build-up of inflammatory neurotoxins such as cytokines that build up after infections such as COVID-19.

So, in long COVID, when this system is back-flowing toxins into the brain, we need to reverse the problem before any attempt is made to stimulate sympathetic activity. This is achieved by the Perrin Technique™. Nitric oxide or a medication that increases sympathetic nervous system activity can only be used safely after the lymphatics are pumping in the correct direction.

The role of the hypothalamus

If one regards any stress factor as an infection, the obvious course of action is to increase the body's defence in staving it off. The fortification of the body is controlled by the autonomic nervous system. The centre of this elaborate web of nerve tissue is primarily found in the hypothalamus and the limbic system of the brain, down to the brainstem, and from the spinal cord spreading throughout the body.

The hypothalamus is a complex bundle of millions of neural networks balancing the functioning of the brain and the rest of the body.

So, the million-dollar question is, where in the hypothalamus should scientists look to uncover the exact problem in long COVID within this small but most multifaceted of all the brain's organs? The answer to this search for the holy grail, I believe, lies in the symptoms and control mechanisms that are affected in this and other similar neuro-lymphatic disorders, such as ME/CFS.

The paraventricular nucleus (PVN) in the anterior superior part of the hypothalamus (see Fig. 28) is probably the most important part of this organ in regulating the neuro-hormonal impact of long COVID, as it has a direct neurological link to the median eminence at the base of the hypothalamus. This is one of the circumventricular organs which have a weak blood–brain–barrier and are gateways into the brain for neuro-inflammatory toxins such as cytokines and serves as an interface between the neural and peripheral endocrine systems. It releases hypothalamic-releasing hormones into the portal capillary bed for transport to the anterior pituitary, which provides further signals to target endocrine systems. The PVN also directly connects with another circumventricular organ – namely, the posterior pituitary, which stores and releases the hormone oxytocin produced in the hypothalamus. This hormone helps childbirth by stimulating uterine contractions and also contractions of breast tissue to aid lactation after childbirth. It is also involved in sexual arousal and has been shown to have a major effect on important aspects of human behaviour such as trust and romantic attachment.

The effects of oxytocin on your brain are highly complex but disturbances in oxytocin levels have been linked to addiction, anorexia, autism spectrum disorder, anxiety and depression plus post-traumatic stress disorder (PTSD) presentations, all of which may show up in one form or another in long COVID patients.

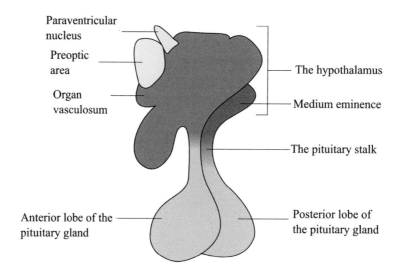

Paraventricular nucleus

Preoptic area

Organ vasculosum

The hypothalamus

Medium eminence

The pituitary stalk

Anterior lobe of the pituitary gland

Posterior lobe of the pituitary gland

Fig. 28 The hypothalamus and the pituitary gland showing the main hypothalamic regions disturbed in long COVID.

Sleep problems

An upsurge in adenosine increases a person's need for sleep, also called the sleep drive or sleep pressure. The sleep drive helps the body maintain sleep-wake homeostasis, or the right amount of sleep and wakefulness over time.

Recent studies have shown that glutamatergic neurons in the paraventricular nucleus (PVN) of the hypothalamus play an important role in wakefulness. It was shown that adenosine can promote sleep by reducing the excitability of PVN neurons. This finding reveals a novel mechanism of adenosine regulating sleep homeostasis.[11]

Scientists at Yale discovered that one of the major functions of the thalamus is the selective control of the flow of sensory-motor information to the cerebral cortex during different states of the sleep-wake cycle and arousal; this is controlled through the actions of various neurotransmitter systems in the brainstem, hypothalamus and cerebral cortex.

University of California's Matthew Walker explains in his book *Why We Sleep* that when the hypothalamus relays messages to the brainstem to power down at night, its influence on the sensory gate of the thalamus stops and we cease perceiving the outside world. The hypothalamus will open the gate again in the morning to wake up the brain.

The neuropeptide produced by the hypothalamus to switch on the brainstem is known as orexin (also known as hypocretin). At night when the hypothalamus stops releasing orexin we fall asleep. This neurotransmitter thus regulates arousal and wakefulness and also has a major control over appetite.[13]

Hypocretin/orexin neurons located in the lateral and posterior hypothalamus control sleep and wakefulness by sending excitatory projections to the brainstem and the locus coeruleus (noradrenaline/norepinephrine), the tuberomammillary nucleus (histamine), and the raphe nuclei (serotonin).

In long COVID, the dysfunctional hypothalamus causes a disturbance in orexin production, switching the brainstem on and off haphazardly, leading to glymphatic drainage problems, disturbed sleep at night and drowsy periods during the day. In severe cases this can lead to the condition narcolepsy.

Professor Matthew Walker's team used MRI scanning to show that a good night's sleep produces a balance between the prefrontal cortex and the amygdala, which is part of the basal ganglia. The prefrontal cortex he describes as our emotional brake and the amygdala as the emotional accelerator. These regions are affected by COVID-19 and resulting pro-inflammatory cytokines as the virus passes through the cribriform plate above the nasal passages through the blood–brain–barrier into the reversed glymphatic system, causing brain fog and concentration problems as well as emotional disturbance.[13]

What happens when we sleep?

There are two types of neurotransmitter involved in the autonomic control of the viscera:

1. The cholinergic neurotransmitters, which use the chemical acetylcholine.
2. The adrenergic neurotransmitters, which use noradrenaline (also known as norepinephrine).

One of the main transmitter substances in the sympathetic nervous system is noradrenaline (also known as norepinephrine). This is formed in the adrenal glands and in a small organ in the brainstem known as the locus coeruleus, which is under the direct influence of the hypothalamus (see Fig. 28).

As mentioned in Chapter 4, research by Xie and fellow scientists at Rochester University, New York, published in 2013, showed that the hypothalamus–locus coeruleus axis is a vital area in the brain for healthy neuro-lymphatic drainage.[14]

I first drew Fig. 28 in 2004 for my doctoral thesis, to show the importance of these two regions in the pathological mechanism leading to ME/CFS, which I believe is as important in the pathophysiology of long COVID. I knew that, since noradrenaline is so important in the functioning of the sympathetic nervous system, this axis must be disturbed in neuro-lymphatic disorders. This is exactly what Xie and his colleagues discovered with their ground-breaking work, showing why we all need restorative delta-wave sleep (see below), as the neuro-lymphatic drainage system occurs mostly during this sleep phase.

In the brain we have around one hundred billion nerve cells (neurons) that are constantly in communication with each other through trillions of connections known as synapses. Brainwaves are produced by synchronised electrical pulses from different areas of neurons communicating with each other.

Brainwaves can be detected using sensors placed on the scalp. They are divided into bandwidths which each have different functions. Slower brainwaves, such as delta-waves, make us feel tired, slow, sluggish, or dreamy. The higher frequencies can create a hyper-alert state, which some call 'wired and fired'. In practice, things are far more complex, and brainwaves reflect different aspects when they occur in different locations in the brain.

Brainwave speed is measured in Hertz (cycles per second) and they are divided into bands delineating them as slow, moderate or fast. The waves are as follows, starting with the slowest:

- delta-waves = 0.5–3 Hz; they occur during deep sleep
- theta-waves = 4–7 Hz; they are present during deep meditation and dreaming
- alpha-waves = 8–13 Hz; they appear during visualisation and meditation
- beta-waves = 14–40 Hz; they are present during wakefulness and REM sleep
- gamma-waves = more than 40 Hz; as with beta-waves, they occur spontaneously during wakefulness and REM sleep.

Recent studies on human sleep have discovered a pumping mechanism in the brain, hitherto unknown, that is produced during … you guessed it … delta-wave sleep. The research team led by Professor Laura Lewis at the Department of Biomedical Engineering at MIT in Boston, USA used MRI scanners to examine 13 healthy young people whilst they slept and found that every 20 seconds a wave of cerebrospinal fluid flows into the brain, replacing a large flow of blood that is stimulated by delta-waves during deep restorative sleep. This extra pumping action of cerebrospinal fluid leads to an increase in pressure within the ventricular system[15] and is most probably the mechanism that improves neuro-lymphatic drainage during delta-wave sleep, as described in the research by Xie and colleagues.[14] Dr Lewis and her team in Boston, have been further examining the neural dynamics that appear during sleep that affect blood flow and the glymphatic system; this is helping us to understand just how important several stages of sleep are for the health of our central nervous system.[16]

A very common symptom of long COVID is unrefreshing sleep. The reason for this is that long COVID patients have too high a level of non-restorative alpha-wave sleep. I will explain this further.

There are five stages of sleep: 1–4 (non-REM sleep) and REM (rapid eye movement) sleep. During these four stages, neurological activity within the brain changes. These stages progress cyclically from 1 to 4 through to REM, then begin again with stage 1. A complete sleep cycle takes an average of 90 to 110 minutes, with each stage lasting between five and 15 minutes.

- Stage 1 is light sleep where you drift in and out of sleep and can be awakened easily.
- In stage 2, eye movement stops, and brain waves become slower, with only an occasional burst of rapid brain waves.
- In stage 3, extremely slow brain waves, called delta-waves, are interspersed with smaller, faster waves. This is deep sleep. It is during this stage that a person may experience sleepwalking, night terrors, talking during one's sleep and bedwetting.
- In stage 4, deep sleep continues as the brain produces mostly delta-waves.

Most patients with long COVID complain that they don't get enough sleep and that when they do, they still feel exhausted. The problem for them is that, though they may often have plenty of sleep, it isn't the restorative delta-wave kind but instead consists of a high proportion of alpha-waves. This is known as 'alpha-wave intrusion'.

The drainage of the brain and spinal cord occurs more during waking hours in long COVID patients, making those patients feel ill and shattered during the daytime. However, during the night, the hypothalamus–locus–coeruleus axis switches on, leading to the 'wired and fired' state, affecting the patient's ability to fall asleep.

During REM (rapid eye movement) sleep, brain waves mimic activity during the waking state. The eyes remain closed but move rapidly from side-to-side, which is often due to brain activity that occurs during dreams. During this phase the rest of the body is immobilised.

It has also been discovered that when dreaming during REM sleep, noradrenaline stops being produced in the brain. This allows a person to replay in the mind traumatic episodes that may have happened recently without the activity of the sympathetic nervous system creating a fear-fight-or-flight response. It is a bit like watching a sanitised movie of the event where you are calm and distant which is a soothing experience for the dreamer. In long COVID the sympathetic nervous system coupled with the lymphatic system of the brain is dysfunctional, so patients often have too much noradrenaline being produced, affecting not only delta-wave sleep but also dreams in REM sleep. So, on top of the fact that most long COVID patients suffer from unrefreshing sleep, they also can experience major anxiety and stress from reliving a traumatic event with all the body's normal reaction to stress in their dream state and the following morning, leading to a state of anxiety.[17]

A technological aid that has just been launched this year may be of real help, as it has been shown to induce more deep sleep and possibly REM dream state. Neuroscientists Dr Alain Destexhe and Luc Foubert of the Paris-Saclay University, have developed a method of converting neural signals into sound sequences, quantifying the wave patterns of the delta-wave signal and generating sound envelopes.

Their research has culminated in the production of the MyWaves Pebble which is a small module attached to the forehead overnight which records the person's own unique brain waves and converts them into music that mimics the waves. The device plays the sounds back, helping patients fall asleep and also stimulating better quality sleep. Since it is a recent invention, at the time of writing this book there are no studies to show that this will definitely help sleep in long COVID but in theory it should.[18]

How the Perrin Technique™ can improve sleep

Hopefully, the Perrin Technique™ is all patients need to restore their healthy sleep, as was seen in a case of a 55-year-old woman who had suffered from COVID-19 in the first wave of the pandemic. In 2020 she was diagnosed in a National Health Service (NHS) clinic as suffering from long COVID. She came to my clinic in Manchester in 2022 and recorded her sleep using a personal monitor that she wore at night (Fitbit). Her symptom severity was scored using the Profile of Fatigue Related States (PFRS) before and after 16 treatments.

The PFRS, as described in Chapter 2, is a multidimensional measure incorporating 54 symptoms associated with disorders such as long COVID. It has four sub-scales: emotional stress, cognitive difficulty, fatigue and somatic symptoms. It was developed by Dr Collette Ray and colleagues at Brunel University, London in 1992 especially to measure the symptoms of these types of illness and evaluate the effects of treatments.[19] It has already been used in the two clinical trials on ME/CFS that I have conducted. Since it is easy to complete and not too difficult to score, it is given to all Perrin Technique™ practitioners to use in their clinics to give a ball-park figure against which to evaluate a patient's progress.

Before her first treatment this patient recorded a PFRS score of 163/324, which is around the 50% severity mark on the symptoms in the week before her consultation, with each of the 54 symptoms scoring 0 for no problem to 6 for very severe. Her sleep waves showed a pre-treatment severe lack of deep sleep, which as we have seen is when delta-waves occur, recording only six minutes throughout the whole night; this was well below normal as it is accepted that adults should generally have an average one to two hours of deep sleep per night.

After her 16th treatment a few months later, her PFRS score had significantly reduced to only 85/324 = 13% severity. Most significantly, her deep sleep had increased to a much healthier 1 hour 6 minutes.[20]

Not only does the type of sleep affect neuro-lymphatic drainage, but it is the position a person adopts during sleep that is also vitally important. A side-lying posture during sleep aids neuro-lymphatic drainage as well as being the best position for the spine in general, placing minimum strain on the spinal joints.[21] Often, I am asked which side is best. Regarding neuro-lymphatic drainage, I don't think it matters that much and I would advise you to start with lying on the side you feel most comfortable on. However, the left side is believed to be the better for improving venous return to the heart and also has been shown to reduce gastric reflux and heartburn.[22]

To maintain a balanced spine in bed, as well as lying on your side, I recommend a small pillow, such as a scatter cushion, placed between your knees throughout the night.

Some patients may develop sleep apnoea, which is when one stops breathing during one's sleep for short periods. This obviously can be dangerous – we need to breathe; so, contact your GP if you think you have this problem. You may need an aid to support breathing at night called a continuous positive airway pressure machine (CPAP), which is the most effective treatment if you have moderate to severe sleep apnoea.

Sleeping pills and low-dose tricyclic antidepressants, such as 10 mg amitriptyline, are prescribed by GPs to be taken an hour before bed. Some patients taking amitriptyline report feeling very drowsy the next morning, so if you have a problem inform your GP. However, sleeping pills don't really help the quality or quantity of sleep. The older drugs such as diazepam were sedatives that dampened the brain but didn't affect the sleep centres. Most of the sleeping pills prescribed today produce a sleep of shorter waves but devoid of delta-waves. As we know, it is the delta-waves that are most important for the glymphatic drainage so sleeping pills leave long COVID patients with more unrefreshing sleep.

The hormone melatonin is important for sleep but melatonin only helps the process of falling asleep, so sometimes this is prescribed by physicians around the world to help ME/CFS patients get off to sleep. However, it doesn't stop restless sleep and doesn't improve the overall quality or quantity of sleep. This is the same as using a SAD lamp for patients who suffer from seasonal affected disorder (SAD), which worsens in the darker winter months and may be the best help in improving the serotonin/melatonin balance by keeping you awake during the day, especially in the winter, and helping you drift off to sleep at a healthier time.

It is best to take melatonin with a time release formula that gradually releases melatonin to your body, to help you stay asleep throughout the night and wake up refreshed. The vitamin B6 taken as part of the B complex that I recommend will help support the production of melatonin.

I also recommend first-generation antihistamines that cause drowsiness one hour before bed, especially for patients with multiple sensitivities, as they often help patients fall asleep.

Talking of medications, some commonly prescribed medicines for heart, blood pressure and breathing difficulties as well as over-the-counter pain killers and cough and cold remedies may have ingredients that disrupt sleep, so if you have disturbed sleep check with your doctor or pharmacist if there is an alternative, better suited medicine.

Other functions controlled by the paraventricular nucleus (PVN)

The PVN connects with the nucleus tractus solitarii which are a pair of cell bodies found in the brainstem, which is a major primary visceral sensory relay station within the brain. The nucleus tractus solitarii receive and respond to stimuli from the respiratory, cardiovascular and gastrointestinal systems under the guidance of messages from the PVN.

The PVN is also the area in the hypothalamus affecting the emotional control of the brain via connections with the amygdala.

As well as the locus coeruleus, another organ located in the brainstem affected by messages to and from the PVN is the parabrachial nucleus of the pons,

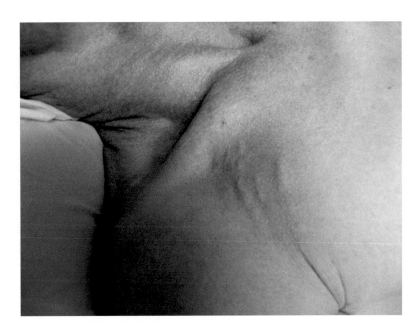

Plate 1: Right subclavicular varicose lymphatics, lacking the bluish hue of varicose veins, in a patient with ME/CFS.

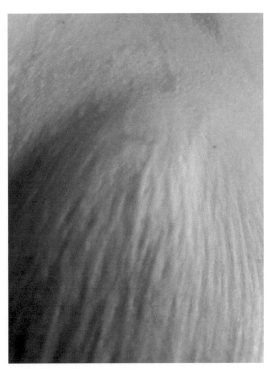

Plate 2: Megalymphatics throughout the left breast of a 73-year-old long COVID patient.

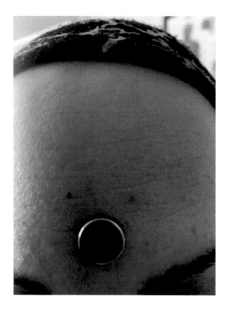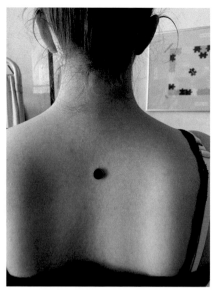

Plate 3: Disc magnets attracted to
(a) forehead of patient and (b) upper/mid thoracic spine.

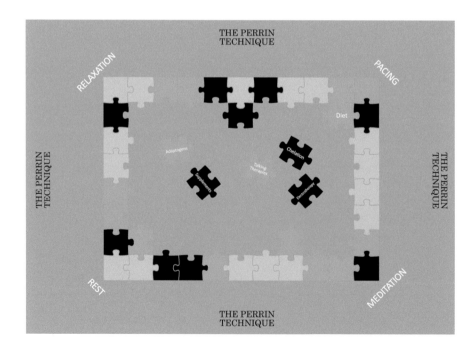

Plate 4: The jigsaw puzzle analogy. Original design
by Ophelia Grace 2023.

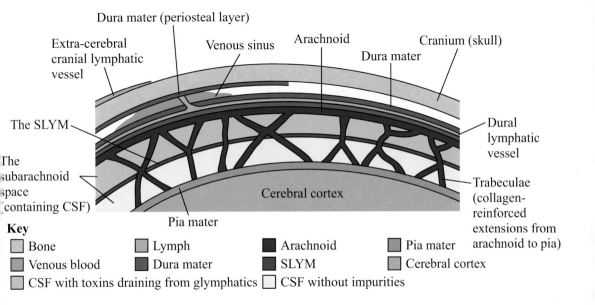

Dura mater (periosteal layer)

Extra-cerebral cranial lymphatic vessel

Venous sinus

Arachnoid

Dura mater

Cranium (skull)

The SLYM

Dural lymphatic vessel

The subarachnoid space (containing CSF)

Cerebral cortex

Trabeculae (collagen-reinforced extensions from arachnoid to pia)

Pia mater

Key

☐ Bone ☐ Lymph ■ Arachnoid ■ Pia mater

■ Venous blood ■ Dura mater ■ SLYM ■ Cerebral cortex

☐ CSF with toxins draining from glymphatics ☐ CSF without impurities

Plate 5: Cross-section of the skull (top) and outer layer of the brain, showing the subarachnoid lymphatic-like membrane (SLYM).

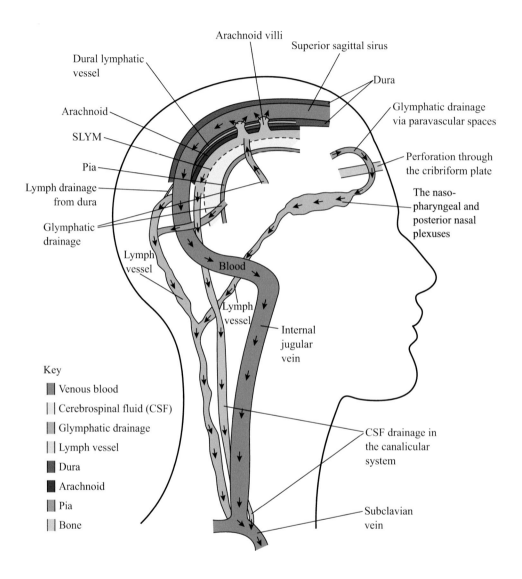

Arachnoid villi

Superior sagittal sirus

Dural lymphatic vessel

Dura

Arachnoid

Glymphatic drainage via paravascular spaces

SLYM

Pia

Perforation through the cribriform plate

Lymph drainage from dura

The naso-pharyngeal and posterior nasal plexuses

Glymphatic drainage

Lymph vessel

Blood

Lymph vessel

Internal jugular vein

Key

- ▮ Venous blood
- ▯ Cerebrospinal fluid (CSF)
- ▮ Glymphatic drainage
- ▯ Lymph vessel
- ▮ Dura
- ▮ Arachnoid
- ▮ Pia
- ▯ Bone

CSF drainage in the canalicular system

Subclavian vein

Plate 6: A schematic diagram showing the key drainage pathways
from the brain.

which relays sensory information such as taste, temperature control and pain, again commonly affected in long COVID.

The pain control mechanisms of the brain in the basal ganglia and thalamus are disturbed in long COVID. This leads to a reduction in the amount of the pain-suppressing neurotransmitter GABA and increased production of the pain stimulant neuropeptide P, which have both been shown to be disturbed when the neuro-lymphatic system becomes dysfunctional.[23]

Also regarding the influence of the hypothalamus on other brainstem activity, it is highly significant that using ultra-high definition 7 Tesla MRI, Thapaliya and colleagues showed visible brainstem anomalies in long COVID patients. Increased brainstem volume was seen in patients suffering more pain, and brainstem volume was less than normal in patients with more respiratory problems.[24]

The PVN has direct influences outside the brain via the parasympathetic vagus nerve and its connections to all the organs of the body, especially the gut, heart and lungs, with spinal sympathetic chain ganglia affecting the control of the lymphatics and the vagus monitoring and controlling the function of all the viscera and blood vessels.

Water balance

Another major hormone in the posterior pituitary regulated by the PVN is vasopressin, also known as the anti-diuretic hormone (ADH), which plays a central role in the water balance of the body. It is secreted if the fluid content of the body becomes highly concentrated and increases the permeability of the kidney tubules reabsorbing water and plays a major role in the maintenance of blood pressure.

Insufficient secretion of ADH leads to excess loss of water and increased thirst, leading in turn to more frequent urination. This is very common in long COVID patients due to an irritation of the sympathetic nerves supplying the bladder, causing further urge to micturate, and also to consume large quantities of water to compensate for the excessive loss of water in urination.

Genetic susceptibility

On page 121 of my PhD thesis published in 2005,[25] I quoted leading ME/CFS expert Dr Jay Golstein (1943–2021): 'Thus CFS/ME, although being a neuro-immune disorder with many differing aetiologies, may actually target genetically predisposed individuals.'[26]

Environmental and genetic factors will alter the rate of chemical metabolism and may predispose an individual to the development of multiple chemical sensitivity. The prognosis of diseases such as ME/CFS will depend on the many factors affecting the body's capability to eliminate toxins.[27]

Mackey suggested that genetically susceptible people with a lower threshold to neuroendocrine stress are more susceptible to a dysfunction of the PVN in long COVID.[28]

Mackey goes on to say: 'In this compromised state, the hypothalamic PVN might then be hyper-sensitive to a wide range of life's ongoing physiological stressors.' This is almost exactly what I claimed was happening with ME/CFS over 30 years ago.

Over-exercising

One such stressor is over-exercise which affects most people involved in top-flight sports. Moderate exercise is generally good for the body, but too much can lead to a build-up of pro-inflammatory cytokines such as IL-6 and TNFα.[29]

Also many sportsmen and women exert more strain upon their dorsal (thoracic) spine in the pursuit of their sport than the average individual. Golf, yachting, cycling and weightlifting are just a few different disciplines that put extra stress on the upper back. Runners also are constantly jarring their spine as they shift all their weight from one leg to the other without both feet on the ground at the same time, which for constant repetitive trauma to the body is much worse than walking, when one doesn't spend any time without one of your feet on the ground. So, in some athletes who may already have a compromised cranial or spinal drainage from genetic causes or previous trauma, their sport could have further irritated the sympathetic nervous system or vice versa with a combination of further trauma affecting the spinal and cranial drainage, often years after they hung up their trainers.

Increased inflammatory cytokines from exertion that drain in the wrong direction would act as catalysts for the immune system to be further compromised. Both scenarios could result in an athlete's susceptibility to the development of long COVID following the infection with the SARS 2 coronavirus.

We now are seeing that, as with ME/CFS, post-exertional malaise is a major symptom of long COVID. Besides intense exercise causing a build-up of lactic acid in muscles, it also causes metabolic acidosis. This metabolic decrease in pH will increase the hormone adenosine in the brain.[30] The opposite effect will occur if there is a decrease in the acidic level which can follow disorders in the regulation of breathing, such as hyperventilation.

As more scientific breakthroughs are made the scientific community will conclude that long COVID is basically ME/CFS in another guise with the same causes and with problems of the hypothalamus being at the root of the illness.

Hyperventilation syndrome (HVS)

The breathing pattern of some long COVID patients resembles that of people suffering from HVS. This syndrome is caused by long-term breathing that is too fast and too heavy. This upsets the balance of oxygen and carbon dioxide in the body. Since the symptoms are so similar, some believe that many cases of long COVID may actually be a form of hyperventilation syndrome.[31]

I feel that sometimes the conditions overlap and some of my patients have HVS as well as long COVID, but they have very different pathophysiology, and patients with this syndrome require much more treatment than just correcting their breathing pattern.

Hyperventilation causes a reduction in carbon dioxide by exhaling more than you inhale, creating more alkaline blood. This leads to a narrowing of the blood vessels and reduces the blood to the brain, leading to cognitive problems and light headedness. The ratio of oxygen to carbon dioxide in the blood is important for the amount of oxygen released to the tissues. Danish physiologist Christian Bohr discovered that without carbon dioxide, oxygen is bound to the haemoglobin in the blood and not released.[32] Consequently, in hyperventilation the lack of carbon dioxide leads to too little useable oxygen.

Therefore, although an increase in oxygen intake is useful in long COVID, too much oxygen without carbon dioxide may be detrimental. So, if one has access to an oxygen tank it is best to use it sparingly, for up to one hour spread over a 24-hour period, and using a rebreather mask that allows the intake of carbon dioxide as well as pure oxygen is preferable.

In cases of hyperventilation, the Buteyko method has been helpful to some of my patients. It is a therapy using specific breathing exercises developed by Ukrainian doctor Konstantin Pavlovich Buteyko in the 1950s and focuses on nasal breathing, breath holding and relaxation methods similar to the exercise that I give on pages 199–203 and in the self-help online video (see page 205).

However, although in cases of hyperventilation syndrome this method might work, one should be very cautious with severe long COVID, so it is not recommended for patients who are very severely ill and bedridden. These patients usually have too little carbon dioxide in their blood (known as hypocapnia) and may improve with rebreather masks and doing Buteyko breathing, but there are many who may just have low oxygen and too much carbon dioxide in their blood (hypercapnia), causing an increase in carbonic acid levels (acidosis) shown as a low pH on blood tests. In such cases, the last thing patients need is more carbon dioxide and they will respond more to just a normal oxygen mask or machines that increase the amount of oxygen in the room. Many patients benefit from using an oxygen concentrator, which is a device that concentrates the oxygen from the air by selectively removing the nitrogen.

The problem of using oxygen as a therapy is that, if one just breathes in oxygen, the increased levels in the blood may exacerbate the oxidative stress, which won't help at all. Oxidative stress has been acknowledged as a common feature in many disease processes. It may induce many of the symptoms of long COVID. In an atom, small negatively charged electrons spin around the central nucleus, akin to planets orbiting the sun. Some atoms have electrons on their outer rings that are shared with other atoms. A group of atoms join to form a larger molecule. A free radical is a molecule with an atom that has lost one of these shared electrons from its outer ring. This will make it highly unstable, and it will damage healthy tissue by trying to obtain another electron from an adjacent molecule. The movement of electrons between chemical species is known as 'reduction' for the electron acceptor and 'oxidation' for the electron donor. Reduction and oxidation always go together and are referred to as 'redox reactions'. Free radicals create problems with healthy redox reactions and can therefore lead to what is known as oxidative stress and, subsequently, many disease processes.

It is, as always with long COVID, complex, and every patient is different so, unless one has access to specialist clinics with labs that can monitor blood oxygen and carbon dioxide balance, one has to be cautious with any breathing therapy.

Antioxidants

As mentioned above, oxidative stress increases free radical production, leading to cell damage and worsening toxicity. Oxygen reacts with free radicals to form peroxidised radicals, which further damage healthy molecules. External factors, such as environmental pollutants and radiation, can lead to major free radical production. Overall, the synthesis of the free radical nitric oxide is increased in long COVID and may be induced by inflammatory cytokines.

Antioxidants restore free radicals to healthy molecules. Antioxidants such as vitamin C have been shown to be major combatants in fighting disease ever since the 1950s when Harman[33] discovered the role of free radicals. The rationale for vitamin C infusion in long COVID rests on the traditional use of megadose vitamin C infusion treatments in autoimmune disease, allergy and a range of other conditions.[34]

As detailed in Chapter 9, I always advise caution when taking any supplements, even vitamin C, as there is a risk of developing kidney stones if the vitamin C intake is too high, so a safe dose that I recommend is up to 500 mg every day. Vitamin C aids calcium absorption, and too much calcium over a long period can lead to kidney stones. Swedish researchers carried out a large study on 23,000 Swedes over an 11-year period and those who reported taking vitamin C supplements were twice as likely to have kidney stones.[35]

Interestingly, this has only been proven to happen in men[36] but I still feel that both men and women should be cautious about overloading vitamin intake and only receive a vitamin infusion from medically-trained practitioners, who can correctly evaluate and reduce any health risks to each individual patient.

Remember that too much of anything, even the good stuff, requires the body to work harder to remove the excess chemicals, whether they be inflammatory toxins, environmental pollutants or vitamins. So, even an excess of vitamin C will lead to more strain on the lymphatics to remove the molecules that are not required. This obviously is not what we wish to achieve so I stress with long COVID, always err on the side of caution, even with vitamins and other supplements.

Neuro-inflammation may also be related to excess oxygen and nitrogen molecules in tissues. This can cause oxidative stress, leading to tissue damage which is discussed above. Adverse effects can occur when nitric oxide (NO) is also affected by oxidative stress. NO is a signalling molecule in many physiological and pathological processes. The free radicals that can lead to oxidative stress can also affect levels of nitrogen availability, leading to many bodily disorders. This process is known as 'nitrosative stress' and has been shown to be a major factor, with oxidative stress, in the build-up of many of the symptoms of ME/CFS, fibromyalgia and long COVID.

Dr Martin Pall, Professor Emeritus of biochemistry and basic medical sciences at Washington State University, maintains that ME/CFS is due to the build-up of nitric oxide (NO) acting through its oxidant form peroxynitrate (ONOO). This NO/ONOO cycle occurs during oxidative stress and creates havoc in all the metabolic pathways in the body, affecting mitochondrial function, increasing inflammation and producing excessive NMDA activity in the brain among many consequences.[37, 38]

The immune system and long COVID

The immune system contains different types of cell needed for innate and specific immune responses. The innate immune system defends the body non-specifically against attack from any source. The defence mechanism that is more specific to the type of infection utilises cells known as lymphocytes. The body provides two basic forms of immune response: humoral (in the body fluid) and cellular (cell-mediated). Both forms are coordinated by the cells of the immune system and their mediators. B-lymphocytes are responsible for humoral immunity and T-lymphocytes are responsible for cell-mediated immunity.

Humoral immunity

Humoral immunity is a specific defence mechanism that involves the production of antibodies, distributed in the blood, lymph and interstitial fluid, which attack foreign antigens throughout the body. It is the major defence mechanism against bacterial infections and utilises circulating antibodies that are produced by specialised B-cells, supported by other cells called T-helper cells (Th cells) which are an important component of the immune system as far as the pathogenesis of long COVID is concerned.

T-helper cells circulate through the blood and lymph nodes for many years and are important in facilitating the activities of other cells involved in immune reactions that destroy invading organisms. T-helper cells can be separated largely into two categories:

- Th1 cells are mainly involved in cell-mediated immunity, as described below, which leads to the activation of T-lymphocytes within specific cells.

- Th2 cells stimulate B-cell activity.

The balance between Th1 and Th2 cells is very important for a healthy immune system. In many disease states there is a dominance of one or the other. For example, Th1-mediated diseases include multiple sclerosis, Crohn's disease of the bowel and lupus (SLE). Diseases that are Th2-mediated include asthma and allergic rhinitis. With long COVID, there is often a disturbed Th1/Th2 balance with both Th1 and Th2 dominance being possible. This is because long COVID affects the central control mechanisms within the brain via the sympathetic nervous system that influences immune regulation.

After recognising foreign material, B-cells multiply rapidly and produce antibodies comprised of large protein molecules known as immunoglobulins. These proteins are produced in large numbers and are usually specific to the infective or foreign agent. The antibodies form complexes with the foreign material and these complexes are then destroyed by other cells, such as macrophages.

Activated B-cells differentiate into plasma cells, which are specialised to synthesise and secrete one to two trillion immunoglobulins, as found in healthy adults.

The immunoglobulins are then divided into different categories, such as IgG and IgM, depending on whether the infection is acute and/or still present. For example, IgG levels indicate that the person has previously suffered from an infection but will often be raised in chronic/long-lasting infections. If there is a long-term co-infection, such as Lyme disease, then the IgG level for the bacterium *Borrelia burgdorferi* will usually be high. Sometimes the immunoglobulin levels are found to be lower than normal, which could indicate an exhaustion of the immune system leading to a susceptibility for some patients with long COVID to pick up any infection going.

Cellular (cell-mediated) immunity

Cellular immunity involves a variety of T-cells that are responsible for protection against viruses, cancers and some disease-causing bacteria, such as *Mycobacterium tuberculosis*. Th cells assist cytotoxic T-lymphocytes (Tc), which actively destroy abnormal cells in disease and malignancies.

A further group of lymphocytes are natural killer (NK) cells, which are part of the body's innate immune system, as mentioned above, and which play an important part in surveying the body for any anomalies and counteracting viral infections and cancer. They possess receptors allowing them to sense and respond to molecular patterns of bacteria, viruses, parasites and fungi, including different types of protein. These NK receptors are known as 'toll-like receptors' (TLRs). They also react to certain environmental toxins.

It has been shown that high amounts of stress or a previous injury can predispose the TLRs to be more sensitive and release inflammatory molecules more readily in response to an immune stressor.[39] The activation of TLRs to the oxidative and nitrosative stress pathways leads to the production of more inflammatory molecules, which creates a vicious circle in diseases such as ME/CFS and long COVID.[40, 41]

Researchers in Iraq have indeed shown that the severity of the immune-inflammatory response during acute COVID-19 may lead to increased nitro-oxidative damage in long COVID.[42]

Scientists in the USA led by Dr Liisa K Selin based in Massachusetts have developed a nebuliser with antiviral, antibiotic, antifungal and anti-inflammatory properties based on their theory that long COVID, like ME/CFS, may be due to an abnormal response to an immunological trigger-like infection, resulting in a dysregulated immune system, specifically the CD8 killer T cells and associated cytokines. What the group has discovered is that a phenomenon known as CD⁺T cell exhaustion is occurring together with a reduction in NK cells. This leads to a condition where persistent antigens that haven't cleared reactivate persistent viruses that remain dormant in the body, especially herpes viruses such as EBV and HHV 6. This causes a massive increase in cytokines and a chronic inflammatory state occurs, placing the body under severe oxidative stress.

Administration of this nebuliser containing antioxidants treats the result of killer T cell abnormalities in the lungs, with potential for the antimicrobial agent to enter the central nervous system and reduce the neuro-inflammation in the brain, helping most of the long COVID symptoms.[43]

Future developments in the Perrin Technique™

Famous sports stars who have developed long COVID include science journalist, author and former runner Gez Medinger, who, together with leading expert immunologist Dr Danny Altman, has written *The long COVID Handbook*[44] which discusses many approaches that have helped this disease. They do acknowledge that the Perrin Technique™ has helped patients but also mention that it may be too expensive for many.

If you shop around, you will find many good practitioners providing my Perrin Technique™ around the world. Those that can afford to pay full price, pay for those that can't. In my clinic in Manchester, I run a sliding scale, and many patients pay reduced amounts if they can't afford the course. There are some practitioners who have huge expenses and running costs due to their locality so the fees in different clinics around the world differ depending on location.

At the moment there is one clinic in the world offering the Perrin Technique™ for free by licensed Perrin Technique™ practitioner, osteopathic physician Dr Ruby Tam DO in Minneapolis, USA. This clinic has been funded by charitable donations which has meant some very fortunate long COVID sufferers in Minnesota can get help without the extra worry of finding the funds for the treatment.

Unfortunately my techniques have not been adopted yet by the National Health

Service in the UK so are all carried out in the private sector. My research colleagues and I aim to carry out a large randomised controlled trial (RCT) with treatment from practitioners as well as self-treatments that will hopefully establish the Perrin Technique™ as part of standard go-to treatments available free in NHS long COVID clinics of the future.

However, before we can try to raise the millions of pounds needed to run a large enough RCT we have first had to undertake a feasibility study to see if patients would engage with and carry out just the home routine. So, last year we carried out a randomised feasibility trial of the Perrin Technique™ self-help intervention to reduce fatigue-related symptoms for patients with long COVID: this was the International Standard Randomised Controlled Trial Number (ISRCTN): 99840264. The details of the self-help regime used in this trial can be found in the next chapter.

Dr Lisa Riste who drove this research forward with her amazing skills and resilience summarises the project, which at the time of writing has just finished but is not yet published.[45]

- Similarities between long COVID and ME/CFS symptoms and an increasing awareness about the debilitating nature of fatigue provided an opportunity to test the Perrin Technique™ self-help intervention.
- Ethical approval for the study was granted by London-Chelsea NHS REC.
- Our feasibility study was promoted by the National Institute for Health and Social Care Research (NIHR) Research for the Future (RftF) team who sent online survey links (Jan–May 2023) on our behalf to their 'database of COVID research volunteers'.
- Participants completed a short initial online survey, with fatigue measured using the Chalder Fatigue Questionnaire (CFQ-11). Those meeting long COVID criteria, without existing reasons for fatigue, were invited to participate and were provided with a Participant Information Sheet and Consent form which was completed over the telephone with one of the research team. This approach alongside

online screening helped us successfully meet our recruitment target of 100 people within five months.

- Participants were randomly allocated to one of two groups: (1) 'intervention' group who used the Perrin Technique™ patient self-help routine immediately OR (2) the 'wait-list control' group who used the same intervention but after waiting 12 weeks.

The intervention comprised self-massage, mobility, flexibility and breathing exercises and 'contrast' (warm/cold) bathing using alternating warm hot-water bottle and gel koolpacks. Participants received a pack containing all the necessary intervention equipment and instructions either immediately or after 12 weeks.

After 12 weeks, participants were sent an email link to complete the follow-up survey, with 79% responding. As this is a feasibility study, we do not have sufficient numbers to formally test if the intervention improved fatigue.

- A reduction (improvement) in CFQ-11 fatigue scores (range 0–33) was observed in both the intervention group (of 4.6 units) and in the wait-list control group (of 2.9 units) after 12 weeks.
- We believe that the self-help intervention in isolation could help support a reduction of fatigue in some people. Further research powered on a larger scale to test for a specific, clinically important, difference in the reduction of symptoms of fatigue (associated with the intervention), potentially either as a standalone, or in conjunction with Perrin Technique™ Practitioners delivering in-person sessions that focus on lymphatic drainage through massage and cranial osteopathy are warranted.
- The feasibility study demonstrated a willingness from patients to participate. Interviews with intervention participants has led to suggested clarification, including presenting the rationale for the various self-help elements and easier access to the self-help online video.[10] On that note, a new Perrin Technique™ self-help video is available online.

Use this QR code to access the Perrin Technique™ Self-help Guide.

As I have said, long COVID patients are diagnosed primarily by the exclusion of other, better understood diseases. However, it is perfectly possible, and common, for people to suffer from more than one disease or disorder at one time. This is why my discovery of physical signs that are common to ME/ CFS, FMS and now long COVID patients is so important, as they provide a much-needed aid in the diagnostic procedure as shown in Chapter 2.

Conclusion

So to answer the initial question in this chapter, 'Can long COVID ever be cured?', this chapter has hopefully shown you that there is no easy answer and the complexities of disturbances in the central nervous system's control, via a dysfunctional hypothalamus, are far reaching.

There is no magic bullet and that is, and will unfortunately remain, the sad truth. However, if one addresses the neuro-lymphatic problem affecting long COVID patients, then many and sometimes all the symptoms reduce. Some fortunate patients will return to a symptom-free state, but not fully cured as they still need to look after their previously weakened neuro-lymphatic drainage.

On a more positive note, some of my early ME/CFS patients have been symptom-free for over three decades after receiving the Perrin Technique™ without the need for any further treatment, so I suppose they would say they were cured.

Chapter 7

Self-help advice

'But the danger was past – they had landed at last,
With their boxes, portmanteaus and bags:
Yet at first sight the crew were not pleased with the view
Which consisted of chasms and crags.'

Lewis Carroll

The Hunting of the Snark

Case: Joe's story

From a very young age I had always been sporty and adventurous. I'd regularly played football my whole life and would always be on the go doing something physical, whether that was my work as a camera operator/filmmaker, or going on hikes, swimming or working out in the gym.

When I first caught COVID-19, in May of 2020, very little was known about the lasting effects it would have on certain people. I was completely unaware that Dr Perrin had already published a paper, warning of the dangers of post-COVID fatigue syndrome (which came to be known as 'long COVID'). I remember speaking to my GP about a month after having COVID-19, telling them that I was collapsing into bed with severe fatigue after going on a short walk around the block, but they told me that it would fade and to carry on exercising… So, I did. Three months on and I was still struggling with an array of symptoms (fatigue being the most debilitating), but there was still very little advice on what was happening to me, it was a very lonely and scary time. I tried to push through and go back to work but I made myself worse and worse until I could not function at all. It was at this point I decided I was going to stop working completely until I was better. At my worst I was bedbound and even getting to the toilet was difficult. I couldn't even get up the stairs.

I first heard about the Perrin Technique™ around two years into my long COVID journey. At that point I had made small improvements due to anti-histamines and pacing, but I was still pretty much house-bound. When I sat down for my initial consultation with Dr Perrin, I instantly felt at ease and had trust in him. It was the first time since being ill with long COVID that I had felt 'heard' and listened to. Everything that Ray said resonated with me and made sense, and he was the first doctor who really understood what I was going through. We went through a full medical history and I scored a 3 on the scale of 1–10. I told him of mild health issues I'd had in the past, and that I was bitten by ticks a year before I got COVID, but didn't get ill or a rash, which resulted in him recommending I get a Lyme disease test. This test proved positive for Lyme and I would never have thought to test for that without his guidance. In hindsight, I recognised that even though I thought I was healthy in the years previous to COVID-19, I wasn't quite right. I would have to sleep on my lunch break at work, and sleep as soon as I got home, and sometimes after playing football or an intense workout I would get aches and fatigue, but it was never bad enough to stop me doing anything, so I took no notice of it. Dr Perrin explained how I had a predisposition for long COVID by confirming I had the physical signs (swollen lymph nodes, varicose lymph, thoracic spinal problems and tenderness at 'Perrin's Point').

Over the next few months I started both Lyme treatment and the Perrin Technique™ simultaneously. Unfortunately, the Lyme treatment didn't quite have the 'curing' effect I'd initially hoped, but I have since realised that all of these treatments, including the Perrin Technique™, are important tools in recovery from long COVID, whether it's been brought on by Lyme, COVID-19, or any other virus etc.

Now, 18 months into my Perrin treatment, I have seen moderate improvements in my symptoms. Before I started the treatment, I barely left the house and had a constant array of different symptoms to deal with; now, although I still have to pace and not push myself, I have much milder daily symptoms and I am able to do much more both physically and mentally. I have recently moved into my first home with my partner and we are soon getting a puppy. These are things I would not have been able to handle before starting this treatment.

During these past 18 months I've been doing various things to help, including brain retraining, vagus nerve stimulation and various medications and supplements, including LDN, hence I could not 100% say which of these treatments has had the most benefit, but I do strongly believe that the Perrin Technique™ is an important tool for those of us who want to recover from long COVID and similar debilitating illnesses.

I now strongly believe that I will make a full recovery, and the Perrin Technique™ is going to continue to be an important treatment in my recovery journey.

Joe Oldroyd, Manchester, UK.
Long COVID patient of Dr Perrin and Licensed Perrin Technique™ practitioner Sylveen Monaghan at the Perrin Clinic, Manchester

Introduction

Osteopathic treatment is not synonymous with manipulation. Many treatments of numerous conditions would be found to be insufficient if they relied on manual therapy alone. As in standard osteopathic practice, advice is given to the patient to help improve their general health. Over the years, it is the patients who have followed my instructions to the letter who have done the best with the Perrin Technique™. This self-help protocol (including the contrast bathing – cold and warm) has been assessed in the major NHS study in the Manchester region described earlier in the book (page 52).

I do realise that the exercises and advice are not always easy to follow, but patients should try their best and will hopefully see the benefit of being strict with the regime. The golden rule regarding exercises for long COVID is the same as with the treatment:

'PAIN = NO GAIN'.

You are doing nobody any favours if you push yourself through the pain barrier. Pain is the body's natural protection, telling you to stop and not to push on. The most important advice that I can give for long COVID is to pace all your activities, mentally and physically, doing half of what you feel capable of doing until you are fully better (see Chapter 5, page 136).

As the treatment improves your health, then gradually increase activity to recondition your body and improve your stamina. However, always stay within the 'half rule' … as I always tell my patients: 'Half of more is still more'.

As explained in Chapter 4, manual treatment improves the function of the thorax and the spine. This is especially so when enhanced by routine mobility exercises. Some effective exercises to improve and maintain the quality of movement of the dorsal spine areas follow. I have described them in easy-to-understand English in the second person as these instructions are important for patients to follow as accurately as possible. (Thanks to Dr Lisa Riste for helping with the plain-language version.)

Dorsal rotation and shrugging exercises

Sitting down, facing ahead (see Fig. 29), place your hands around both sides of your neck with thumbs nearest your shoulders, elbows facing forward and down. Slowly rotate your upper body, first to the right (from the waist up) keeping your head and neck facing the same direction as your upper body. This gentle rotation is designed not to stretch muscles and joints, but gradually and subtly to increase movement of your upper back. You should only rotate or twist about 45 degrees in total from right to left. Now twist gently and slowly, without stopping in the middle, to the left side. The movement must be rhythmic and as relaxed as possible during the entire process. This should be repeated five times each way.

In the next exercise (see Fig. 30), while sitting, cross your arms and hug your shoulders with your hands. Then rotate your back five times each way through an arc of 45 degrees. Make sure that your head, neck and shoulders all stay in line with each other. This exercise encourages movement in the middle section of the thoracic spine.

Finally, in the third exercise (see Fig. 31), still sitting, fold your arms at your waist. Slowly rotate your back five times each way, again keeping your head, neck and shoulders in line. This exercise improves mobility of the lower thoracic spine.

Following the above three exercises, stand up if you are able, and gently roll your shoulders slowly forward five times and then slowly backwards, repeating the rolls five times (see Fig. 32).

The three-stage trunk rotations together with shoulder rolls will take about one minute, if done at the correct speed.

You should carry out the entire sequence of rotation and shoulder rolling three times a day. Since it is a very gentle exercise, even if your ME/CFS is severe, this should not prevent you from carrying out these exercises. However, you are advised to cease exercises if pain develops at any time during or following the routine.

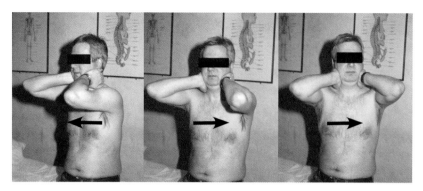

Fig. 29 Upper thoracic rotation exercise.

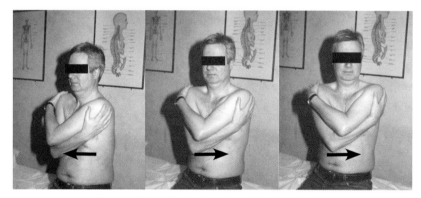

Fig. 30 Mid-thoracic rotation exercise.

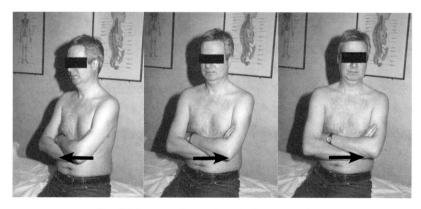

Fig. 31 Lower thoracic rotation exercise.

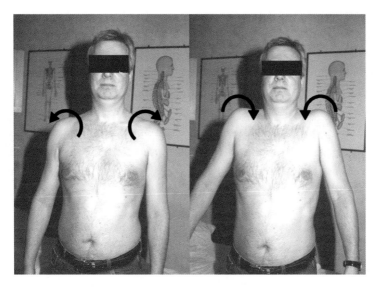

Fig. 32 Shoulder rolling exercise.

Home-massage routine

Patients are also advised to aid the lymphatic drainage of their head and spine through a self-massage routine carried out at home which further aids lymphatic drainage from the central nervous system into the blood. As we now know, the main bulk of toxins are drained from the brain into the lymphatics during deep delta-wave sleep (see page 96), which is why delta-wave sleep is so restorative. However, we now know that long COVID patients unfortunately don't get much delta-wave sleep but too much alpha-wave sleep, which is non-restorative and leads to hyperarousal of the sympathetic nervous system in the brain.

Therefore, stimulating neuro-lymphatic drainage at night will hopefully mimic what is meant to happen naturally and you will wake up more refreshed as the toxins drain out of your central nervous system, especially as the bulk of delta-wave naturally occurs in the first few hours of sleep. So, the full routine as shown below should be done once in the evening, preferably just before bedtime.

Nasal release

Sitting down, rest your elbows on a table in front of you and apply gentle pressure with the pads of both index fingers to just below where the upper and lower eyelids meet (in the corner of your eyes). Push slightly upwards or, if more comfortable, pull slightly downwards just above the bridge of your nose (see Fig. 33). Choose the position that feels most comfortable and lets you breathe the easiest. If neither method is more effective at aiding breathing, then you should always choose downward pressure as the default method. For the first 10 days of this self-treatment, apply this pressure for 7 minutes.

After the first 10 days, you should continue with nasal release for a 1-minute period each day in order to maintain the improvement.

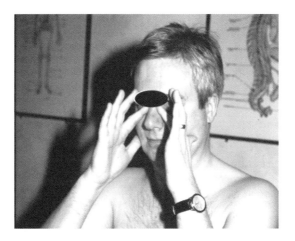

Fig. 33 Nasal release.

Facial massage

Spread the fingers of one hand across your face, as if trying to span your forehead, and slowly stroke your fingertips down your face to your chin (see Fig. 34). Repeat this gentle facial stroking for 20 seconds with one downwards stroke roughly every 4 seconds.

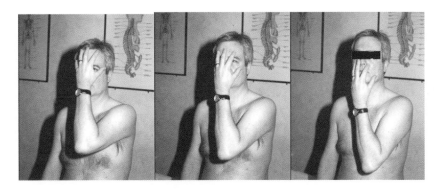

Fig. 34 Facial self-massage.

Head massage

You should now gently massage the sides and back of your head:

1. For the sides of your head: repeat the strokes used in the facial massage above, using your hands to gently stroke downwards on both sides of your head at once, from the top of your head to your chin, with the same slow rhythm again for 20 seconds (see Fig. 35).

2. For the back of your head, repeat again with gentle downward stroking using both hands at the back of your head working down to your neck for a further 20 seconds.

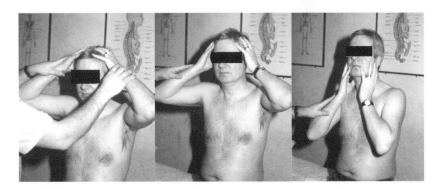

Fig. 35 Self-massage to head.

For the remainder of the self-massage, you should use some massage oil to avoid friction. As I said earlier (page 104), this can be sweet almond oil, coconut oil or similar depending on any allergies or sensitivities you may have. NB: Avoid baby oil or any other petrochemical-based cream. Recently, I was visiting a patient who came up with an alternative for those who wish to remain cream and oil free. He has been using a large soft bristle make up brush that is usually used to apply a blusher. This provides the correct amount of pressure with little friction and so is an acceptable alternative when carrying out self neck and breast massage. However, one should occasionally do the breast massage with hands so that one can detect any changes that could occur, such as cysts and lumps that may need further investigation.

Self-massage to front of neck

Lie down and, using the oil, massage gently from the top of your neck just under your ear, down towards your collarbone using the back of your fingertips for 20 seconds on each side (see Fig. 36).

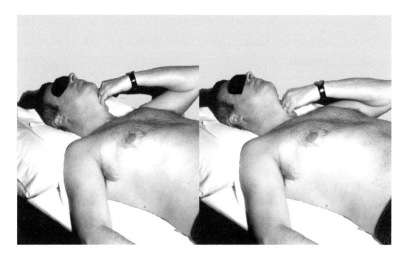

Fig. 36 Self-massage to front of neck.

Breast massage

The breast/chest massage is easiest done in three sections (outer, centre and inner), using massage oil, for 20 seconds in each area so the right and left areas are massaged for 1 minute each. The massage must always be towards the clavicles, thus directing the lymph away from the axillary (armpit) lymph nodes to avoid risk of glandular swelling in the armpits (see Fig. 37).

• Outer: Massage the side of your chest with a slow rhythmic stroking movement, with the flat fingertips of one hand and rubbing upwards with the other hand in a loose fist position. Start just underneath the breast area and work upwards towards the collarbone (not towards the armpits).

• Centre: Repeat the massage movements but working over the centre of the breast so the massage is up over the nipple area, again up to the collarbone.

• Inner: This is the same movement but using the backs of the fingers with both hands flat on the inside area of the chest.

In Fig. 37, the black arrow shows the direction of the self-massage technique. The pressure applied by the patient should be much less than during a treatment session, concentrating only on the superficial lymphatics.

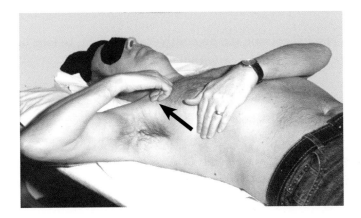

Fig. 37 Self-massage of the breast.

Back massage

Having adopted a prone position, the patient receives back massage from a family member or friend. The massage routine comprises of 1 minute of gentle upward effleurage to the sides of the spine, finishing in the shoulder region, level with the clavicles. If no help is available, patients should use back brushes to accomplish the back massage. There are specific back massagers made out of wood with rubber heads, or other metal ones which are extendable and rubber rollers. Both these massage hammers are easy to use and are available to buy online. One useful tool to do the back massage for oneself is a small fluffy paint roller with a long handle used to paint behind wall radiators. Just move the roller upwards each side of the thoracic spine to the level of the collar bones just below the base of the neck.

Back of neck massage

The self-massage routine ends with slow downwards rhythmic massage of the back of the neck towards the level of collarbone carried out for 20 seconds on each side of the spine.

The full routine

The full routine is summarised in Table 7.1.

Table 7.1 The full routine (to be completed at night, before bed, by the patient or with help from a carer)

Nasal release	Rest elbows on table; place tips of index fingers on either side of nose (above the bridge); gently pull down/press up for 7 minutes for the first 10 days, followed by 1 minute thereafter
Facial massage	With fingers spread out apply a little pressure and gently stroke down the face for 20 seconds (five times taking 4 seconds each)
Head massage	a. Gently stroke down the sides of the head, for 20 seconds each side

	b. Gently stroke down the back of the head for 20 seconds with both hands
Front of neck massage (use oil)	Lying down, massage gently from top of neck just under ear down towards collarbone using back of fingertips for 20 seconds on each side
Breast massage (use oil)	Up for 1 minute each side (NB Divide breast into three sections; outer, middle and inner and massage for 20 seconds each towards the collar bone and not the armpit)
Back massage (use oil)	Up for 1 minute each side of the spine (careful not to touch spinal column)
Back of neck massage – back (use oil)	Down for 20 seconds each side (simultaneously or one and then the other, whichever you find best)

Some patients whose symptoms are not too severe may find that a more regular self-massage routine speeds up the healing process. In the following extra top-up routine, only the head and neck are targeted, and it starts with the nasal release for only 1 minute. The shorter self-massage routine is completed with downward massage of the face and head followed by gently stroking down the front and back of the neck. This can be done anywhere as it is achieved without oil and without having to remove any clothing (see Table 7.2).

Table 7.2 The head and neck drainage routine (to be completed up to three times a day – only for patients who have minor symptoms)

Nasal release	For 1 minute
Facial massage	Down for 20 seconds at a time
Head massage	Down for 20 seconds at a time, sides and back
Neck massage	Down for 20 seconds at a time each side, front and back

Other useful additional exercises

Cross-crawl

One can stimulate both halves of the brain to work together in harmony with the whole body by the following simple exercise known as the cross-crawl. The cross-crawl exercise is basically marching on the spot crossing one limb over to the opposite side. The marching action should be slow and deliberate, with your right arm moving in unison with your left leg, with best results achieved by touching your flexed left knee with your right hand.

This action is repeated moving your left arm forward together with your right leg, touching your right knee with your left hand. ME/CFS patients sometimes find this simple task difficult to perform at the beginning of therapy, since their bodies are so un-coordinated. It is very important not to move the arm and leg of the same side together, as this will succeed in throwing your body (and mind) further out of balance.

After practising for a while, patients are able to carry out the cross-crawl exercise without too much difficulty. The marching routine is to be done for up to 5 minutes during an entire day, a minute or so at a time. Remember that it shouldn't exhaust you as any exercises that over-exert you will worsen your condition and are always to be avoided.

This technique can be adapted by very severely affected patients who are wheelchair-bound or even bedridden. This can take the form of the patient gently moving their left hand slowly up and down together with their right foot followed by their right hand together with their left foot and flexing and extending each hand and foot five times at a time. This can be repeated every day, or more frequently if the patient feels that they are still following the 'half rule' without ever exhausting themselves.

Strengthening exercises for hypermobile spinal joints

Suboccipital hypermobility

Many long COVID patients suffer from a comorbidity of joint hypermobility. This may be hereditary, and part of the condition known as Ehlers-Danlos syndrome (see Chapter 2). Some patients suffer from a weakness at the very top of the spine known as suboccipital hypermobility/cranio-cervical instability. I advise the following isometric exercise routine (i.e. with pressure only, but no actual movement). It is essential that no movement of the neck takes place. Repeat the six different stages of the exercises five to 10 times as long as it is not too taxing for you. The whole routine (below) should be completed three times a day as long as you can cope with the exercises and feel that it is not too strenuous. In other words, keeping with the tenet of the 'half rule', you should feel that you are easily able to do double the amount of exercise without aggravating your symptoms.

1. Lying down or sitting upright, gently hold one or both hands on your forehead. Try to slightly flex your neck, i.e. face looking downwards, but stop any movement with your hands pressed on your forehead so that your head remains at all times facing forward. This attempt to bend your head downwards should be maintained for 3 seconds and then you should gently relax the pressure before repeating the exercise five to 10 times in total (see Fig. 38a).

2. Next try to slightly extend your neck (i.e. bending head back), again without any actual movement, stopping the extension with your hands pressed on the back of your head (occiput). This attempt to bend your head backwards should be maintained for 3 seconds and then you should gently relax the pressure before repeating the exercise five to 10 times in total (see Fig. 38b).

3. Try to slightly tilt your head to the right, stopping any movement with your right hand on the side of your head. This attempt to bend your head sideways should be maintained for 3 seconds and then you should gently

relax the pressure before repeating the exercise five to 10 times in total (see Fig. 39a).

4. Repeat the same exercise in stage 3 for the left side (see Fig. 39b).

The first four stages gently strengthen the whole neck; however, the next two exercises are specifically designed to remedy the suboccipital instability.

5. Now try to slightly flex the very top of your neck by trying to tuck in your chin, stopping any movement with both your thumbs pressed into the inside of your chin. This attempt to tuck in your chin should be maintained for 3 seconds and then you should gently relax the pressure before repeating the exercise five to 10 times in total. For the exercise to be successful it is important that little or no movement of your chin or neck takes place (see Fig. 40a).

6. Try to slightly extend the very top of your neck by trying to poke out your chin, stopping any movement with one or both hands pressed against the front of your jaw (see Fig. 40b). This attempt to push out your chin should be maintained for 3 seconds and then you should gently relax the pressure before repeating the exercise again five to 10 times in total. As with stage 5, it is essential that little or no movement of your chin or neck takes place.

Note: The white arrows in Figs 38–40 represent the direction of resistance offered by your hands.

Hypermobility of the lower lumbar region

In cases of hypermobility of the lower lumbar region, I advise patients to carry out the following exercise routine. You should repeat the different stages of the exercises up to 10 times, three times a day, as long as it is not too taxing for you.

1. First, lie on your back, preferably on a firm surface such as a yoga mat, with knees bent. Lying on the bed will be okay if you find it difficult to

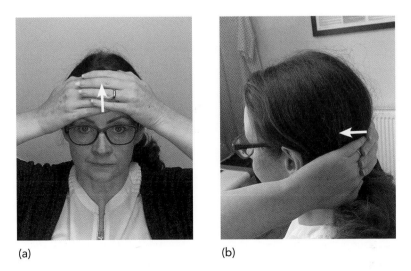

(a) (b)

Fig. 38 Cervical isometrics: (a) Attempting to bend head forward, prevented by gentle backwards pressure of hands; (b) Attempting to bend head back, prevented by gentle forward pressure of hands.

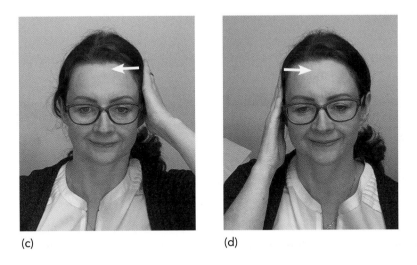

(c) (d)

Fig. 39 Cervical isometrics: (a) Attempting to bend head to the left, prevented by gentle counter-pressure of left hand; (b) Attempting to bend head to the right, prevented by gentle counter-pressure of right hand.

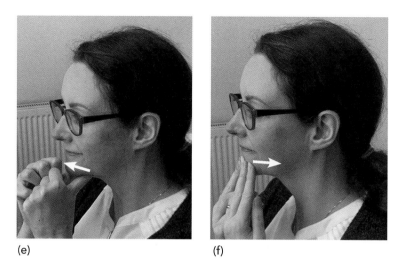

(e)   (f)

Fig. 40 Cervical isometrics: (a) Attempting to tuck in chin, prevented by gentle forward counter-pressure of thumbs; (b) Attempting to push chin forward, prevented by gentle backwards counter-pressure of fingers.

lie on the floor.

2. Next, lift your bottom and lower back gently up a few centimetres from the floor and hold for 3 seconds.

3. Slowly lower your bottom and gently relax the muscles before repeating the exercise. For those familiar with yoga, this exercise is similar to 'the bridge' position but without lifting the bottom so high.

Active head rest

This is a do-it-yourself technique that I recommend for patients if I feel that the cranial flow could do with a little extra help, usually in the later stages of the treatment programme, as initially it may be too much too soon. It should only be done by patients at the beginning of therapy if they cannot access the actual Perrin Technique™ treatment. As we only used at home self-treatment techniques in the NHS study, active head rest was included in the trial but if the patient is having cranial treatment this is not required in the early part of the treatment programme. It is a simple exercise that is also taught by practitioners of the Alexander technique.

In the early days of osteopathy in the late 19th century, Dr Andrew Taylor Still, the founder of osteopathy, developed a similar exercise when he suffered from a severe headache. The story goes that he lay down and balanced his head on a swing. In those days in Missouri standing swings that rested just above the ground were all the rage, and Taylor Still found that by positioning his head at a certain angle he felt comfortable and in a short time his headache disappeared. This probably was the first cranial treatment ever performed.

One of the principles taught to me as a student osteopath was 'comfort governs function', which basically means that if the body is in the most comfortable position it will function better. So, if the head is positioned in the most comfortable position then the cranial flow, AKA the neuro-lymphatic drainage from the brain, will improve. Nowadays we don't use planks of wood or swings. You, the patient, should experiment with a paperback book or books placed under your occiput, which is the bone at the back of the head, until the most comfortable angle is achieved (see Fig. 41). You should lie on a yoga mat or a duvet placed on the floor, so the ground is firm but not too hard, in a semi-supine position (on your back with knees bent) for about 10–15 minutes at night, preferably after the self-massage routine summarised in Table 5.1, just before going to sleep.

If you do not find any suitable book that you feel comfortable with, then this exercise should not be carried out as it will probably worsen the condition. It only works if it feels comfortable … remember: 'comfort governs function'.

Breathing exercises

COVID-19 was identified early on as a similar virus to severe acute respiratory syndrome (SARS) that affected the lungs of many people in Hong Kong and

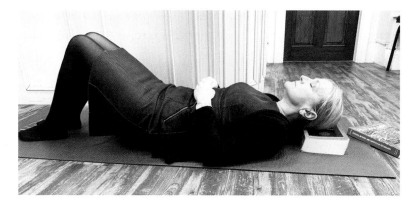

Fig. 41 Active head rest.

Canada in 2003. It was initially termed SARS-CoV-2 and the focus of most of the treatment for the acute patients was to help their breathing. Many of the survivors were left with residual respiratory problems as well as having the post-acute sequelae that we now call long COVID.

So, on top of all the treatment and advice mentioned in this book to aid lymphatic drainage of the brain and the spine, I often give some gentle exercises to aid respiratory mechanics and improve the breathing of the patient.

Rib stretch and diaphragmatic exercise

This sitting exercise was given to all the patients on the long COVID NHS feasibility study into the self-treatment and exercise routines that are part of the Perrin Technique™. It was well-tolerated and has always been part of my armoury when treating any patient with respiratory problems, whether it be asthma or chronic bronchitis; this simple exercise will help open the thorax and aid better expansion of the lungs.

The patient should begin by sitting with their hands on either side of their neck and their back upright (do not clasp the fingers at the back).

1.   The patients should breathe out through their nose whilst bending their head,

neck and back forward and down, with the elbows closing in on each other.

2. The patient should hold this pose with back bent forward and head down for 3 seconds before breathing in.

3. When breathing in through the nose the patient should open their elbows pushing them forward and out whist still holding the sides of their neck and at the same time lifting their head up, extending the spine until the elbows are out to the side as far as possible at full inhalation.

Immediately breathe out and repeat stages 1, 2 and 3 for 10 cycles, three times a day.

This routine should be done slowly and should not cause any pain to the neck, back, shoulders or elbows but it is essential to hold for 3 seconds when in full exhalation to avoid the patient hyperventilating and keeling over.

In health journalist James Nestor's best-selling book *Breath*,[1] there are plenty of breathing techniques to improve overall health including certain ones that help the autonomic nervous system work better, such as alternative nostril breathing, but the two I feel can help patients most are Buteyko breathing and once the neurolymphatic system works better try humming to increase the levels of nitric oxide for 5 min a day.

Additionally the following breathing techniques can also help overall health.

- **Buteyko breathing technique:** In the 1950s Ukrainian doctor Konstantin Buteyko developed many breathing techniques that all use breath retention exercises to control the speed and volume of breathing, extending the time between inhalation and exhalation in line with the body's metabolic needs. The basic technique involves comfortably holding the breath for a few seconds after exhaling before inhaling slowly and gently and repeating the cycle up to 500 times a day, always breathing in through the nose if possible, which will humidify, warm and clean the incoming air.

- **Humming:** Many long COVID patients suffer from pain and inflammation

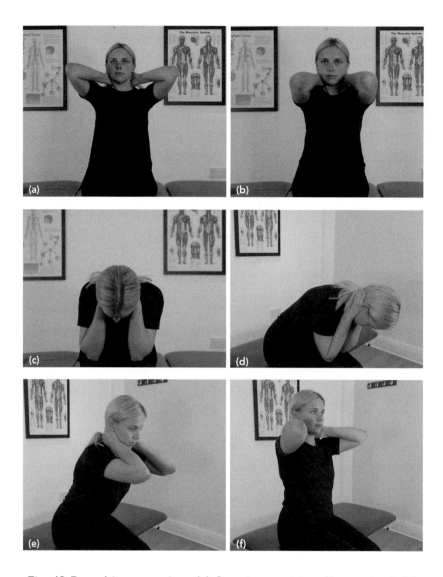

Fig. 42 Breathing exercises (a) Starting position (front view) (b) Patient, whilst breathing out, bending forwards, elbows closing in (front view) (c) Patient in bent sitting position (front view) (d) Patient in bent sitting position (side view) (e) Patient breathes in, straightening back whilst pushing elbows out (side view) (f) Patient back at the starting position (side view).

in their sinuses. Many have over the years suffered from chronic sinusitis long before their present illness. Humming any song whilst breathing, even for just a few minutes a day, causes the air to oscillate which speeds up the exchange of air between the sinuses and the nasal cavity. It has been shown to improve health by leading to an increase in the levels of nitric oxide (NO) produced in the sinuses.

Once the lymphatics are working better in the correct direction, an increase in nitric oxide may help long COVID as it is known to have antiviral properties and to increase oxygenation. It also relaxes the smooth muscles of the blood vessels by acting as a neurotransmitter in the brain that can modulate levels of sympathetic nerve activity and thereby blood pressure as well as the smooth muscles of the lymphatic collecting vessels. So, a healthy increase of NO will aid circulation in the blood and help drainage in the lymph. One study showed that if you can increase the intensity and length of the humming to 1 hour a day, it may help chronic sinusitis in just a few days. However, nitric oxide is a free radical that can lead to cell and tissue damage when taken in excess so care should be taken not to overload your nitric oxide levels … balance is the key to everything.[2, 3]

Swimming

The best rehabilitative activity for the recovering long COVID patient is a swimming stroke known as adapted back sculling (see Fig. 43), which is done lying on the back and gently wafting the arms along just beneath the water surface, slowly propelling you backwards; however, with this rehabilitative exercise you should slowly move your legs up and down as well.

Avoid breaststroke as this is just wrong on so many levels. When I was specialising in sports injuries, the top-level swimmers that I saw most were the breaststroke swimmers. This is the most common stroke among casual swimmers but places unnatural strain on the neck, shoulders, spine, pelvis, hips and knees … besides that, it's okay.

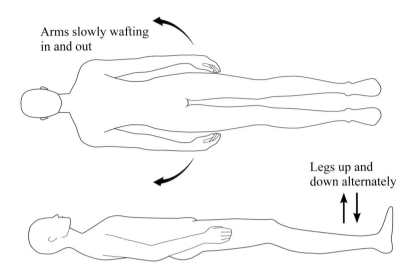

Fig. 43 Adapted back sculling technique.

As you are able to do more, then you can introduce backstroke and front crawl but try not to break any speed and distance records. One of my patients once threw caution to the wind and as soon as she felt able to swim a few lengths she decided to swim a couple of kilometres and spent the next few months in bed, recovering. Swimming in a saltwater pool, if one is available, or the sea if it is not too cold, is preferable to a chlorinated pool due to the toxic effects of the chlorine, especially if you also have been diagnosed as suffering from mast cell activation syndrome or multiple chemical sensitivity.

Conclusion

One of the most important things I have learned in the past 35 years, after seeing thousands of patients improve with the treatment plan, is that those patients who do the best follow the relevant instructions given in this chapter implicitly. None of the routines and exercises should ever hurt . Remember the golden rule: PAIN = NO GAIN. Also stick to the 'half rule' – i.e. always do 50% of what you feel capable of, so, if the above instructions are too much, reduce the timings of the technique to what you feel comfortable doing whilst staying within safe parameters.

The official free online video guide is available for all on the Perrin Technique™ website – just scan the QR code below. Please use this visual guide, if you are able, at the beginning of your recovery journey together with treatment from a trained licensed Perrin Technique™ practitioner, if possible. Although there are other videos online with my techniques, there are some that give advice that I have not sanctioned and don't agree with. The information in this chapter and the video guide are to show you exactly how these exercises should be safely done to achieve the best results.

Use this QR code to access the Perrin Technique™ Self-help Guide.

Chapter 8

Other treatments that may help

'In my youth said the sage', as he shook his grey locks, 'I kept all my limbs very supple. By the use of this ointment – one shilling the box – allow me to sell you a couple?'

Lewis Carroll

Alice's Adventures in Wonderland

Case: Anna's story – The Perrin technique™: the key that unlocked my recovery from long COVID

Reflecting on my experience of long COVID, I probably need to return to my school days to identify the beginning of my story. I was an academic high achiever, more by dint of hard work than genius, and I have always thrown myself 100% into what I do. By the time COVID-19 hit the UK in 2020, I was happily married with three children and a part-time teaching job, a three-generation household and a busy social life. I think I was always tired! My father, who lived with us, died at home of leukaemia in April 2020; I helped my mother nurse him at the end and then we all muddled through grief in lockdown. It was a relief to return to our normal routines.

I contracted COVID-19 in November 2021, with mild symptoms – and then struggled with persistent fatigue afterwards. I just didn't 'bounce back'. I pushed through for 11 months until I had a breakdown in October 2022. By then I had anxiety linked to the pressures of living with fatigue, and I was completely drained and overwhelmed. I couldn't think straight or stop crying. I thought perhaps a couple of days off work would help … It turned into six months.

NHS rehabilitation was supportive but offered nothing to help me improve my condition. I was given mental health support and tips on pacing which reassured me that I was doing the right thing but gave me no hope of recovery. I started to wonder if it was all in my mind. Maybe everyone felt like this, and I was just weak? It was a long, dark winter.

After a recommendation from a friend, I was assessed by Rakhee Mediratta at her Chalfont clinic and started the Perrin Technique™ at the end of January 2023. Within three weeks of starting treatment, I had an hour one evening when I felt well again, like myself! It made me realise how physically unwell I was, how it wasn't in my mind – and this gave me hope that I could get better. Rakhee had accurately predicted this, and as time and treatments progressed, I have felt increasingly well for longer periods of time, just like she said I would.

An early revelation for me was the connection between past stress and the onset of long COVID. I had always wondered if somehow the death of my father was a contributing factor in my illness and here at last was a physiological explanation. The metaphor of a blocked toilet springs to mind – put too much stuff down the loo and eventually the flushing mechanism stops working! The stress of the COVID-19 infection had pushed my already overloaded system to breaking point.

I committed myself fully to the work of recovery. I attended weekly appointments and followed the daily program of warm and cold compresses, rotation exercises, self-massage and supplements as closely as I could. I also worked on optimising the 'corner pieces' of the jigsaw puzzle of health and recovery: sleep, diet, stress reduction and rest. It was a huge investment of time, money and effort – but I knew after that first glimpse of my old self that it was worth it.

If you have a chronic condition or support someone who has one, I imagine you know how hard it can be mentally, as well as physically. Rakhee's expertise was a big part of holding me steady as I worked on my recovery. Seeing her weekly for the Perrin Technique™ gave me a sense of being guided and supported through what amounted to a fundamental shift in my identity and sense of self. In this way as well as physically, the Perrin Technique™ has been transformative.

Now, 15 months on, I only have pockets of time when I feel unwell if I have been busier or more stressed than usual. I recently experienced a whole day when I was completely symptom free. I feel good, and I enjoy life again. It's true that I do less now than I did before COVID-19, but I experience it more fully. Long COVID feels like a blessing in disguise, as it has taught me how to slow down, set boundaries without guilt and enjoy life moment to moment instead of always striving to accomplish more – and the Perrin Technique™ was the key that unlocked my recovery. I currently still limit my activity, I often rest during the day, and I maintain the evening massage routine. I have the Perrin treatment every four to six weeks. Rahkee's advice as I transition back towards 'normal' life is invaluable, and she continues to guide me towards finding a healthy balance between rest and activity. I am so grateful to Dr Perrin, Rahkee and her colleagues for their support and expertise in a condition that so few doctors seem to understand.

Anna Taylor, Buckinghamshire, UK, May 2024
Patient of Licensed Perrin Technique™ practitioner Rakhee Mediratta

The Alexander technique

The Alexander technique is a teaching programme based on postural balancing that helps you change long-standing habits that cause unnecessary tension in the body. It was discovered in the 1890s by an Australian actor, Frederick Matthias Alexander, who initially developed what he called 'the work' to help his vocal problems.

An Alexander teacher will help you learn how to improve your health via the natural balance of your head, neck and back, what Alexander called 'the primary control'. The technique works through re-establishing this natural balance to promote easy upright posture and improved functioning of the body and mind.

It may not be that much of a coincidence that it developed just after osteopathy officially came into being in 1885 as many concepts of Alexander's are very osteopathic in nature, including the active head rest (page 198) which is part of the self-treatment strategies I have advised for long COVID since their inception in 2020 and which was part of the NHS self-management research project my team at the University of Manchester undertook in 2023.

My own clinic in Manchester had a wonderful Alexander Teacher, Miriam Press, who worked alongside my osteopathic and physiotherapy colleagues, helping many patients with ME/CFS and fibromyalgia until her death a few years ago.

As a way of continuing any postural improvement gained from the Perrin Technique™, on top of the exercises given by the practitioner, long COVID patients are encouraged to seek a local Alexander teacher if they have any ongoing postural problems or just to maintain the balance. According to an article published last year in the *Archives of Physical Medicine and Rehabilitation*, classes in Alexander technique teach you ways to connect your brain with your movement and can bring flow, balance, lightness and ease into your daily life, and may help in reducing fatigue and brain fog.[1]

Yoga

Recovered ME/CFS patient Fiona Agombar has taught therapeutic yoga in London since 1999. Her book *Beat Fatigue with Yoga*[2] has some excellent techniques that may help.

Fiona claims, quite rightly, that yoga can help ME/CFS, and so in many patients with long COVID her techniques may help. Some of the reasons for the benefits of yoga she gives are listed below.

1. It calms the nervous system, especially through relaxation exercises.
2. It uses meditation, relaxation and visualisation exercises that help increase slow brain waves, calming the sympathetic nervous system.
3. It reduces stress.
4. It increases cognitive function.
5. It helps in the transport of oxygen and oxygenation of tissues.
6. It aids detoxification.
7. It improves the functioning of most bodily systems.
8. It increases energy.

All of the above are relevant and important in long COVID so gentle yoga practices may be helpful. However, one has to be very careful not to put too much pressure on the upper spine so in any exercise activity, whether it be yoga, tai'chi or pilates, patients have to listen to their body and the golden rules with any activity based approach **less is more** and **pain equals no gain!**

Posture and ergonomics

You should avoid slumping into a soft chair. When relaxing, you should sit in a supportive chair and, if your long COVID is severe, aim to lie on your side as much as possible on a couch or a bed with your head well supported and a pillow between your knees. Lying on your side puts minimal strain on to your spine. It has also been shown that neuro-lymphatic drainage occurs more when lying on the side and that a lateral sleeping position is the best position to most efficiently remove waste from the brain.[3]

As I have said elsewhere in this book, I am often asked which side is best. Regarding neuro-lymphatic drainage, I don't think it matters that much and I would advise you to start with lying on the side you feel most comfortable on. However, the left side is believed to be the better for improving venous return to the heart and also has been shown to reduce gastric reflux and heartburn.[4]

However, even severely affected patients should spend some time attempting to sit up if possible, as gravity will aid the newly discovered flow of cerebrospinal fluid into the bloodstream via a pair of canals in the neck (see Chapter 6). If raising the head is impossible, then it is of great importance that the patient or their carer massages down the front sides of the neck at least three times a day as shown in Fig. 36 (Chapter 7).

Far infrared (FIR) saunas

A FIR sauna heats your body directly via infrared waves on the far end of the light spectrum as opposed to a traditional sauna that uses heat to warm the air around your body. An infrared sauna stimulates sweating and increases heart rate at lower temperatures than does a regular sauna.

Several studies have shown some evidence that using an infrared sauna is beneficial in the treatment of chronic health problems, such as high blood pressure and Alzheimer's disease. The gentle warming process of the whole body stimulates more parasympathetic activity whilst reducing sympathetic overloading, leading to increased β-endorphins and relaxation.[5] FIR has also been shown to improve heart and lung function, helping endothelial cells.

Researchers from Kagoshima University in Japan have developed a specific treatment known as Waon therapy using FIR saunas that may be beneficial. The process is carried out for two to six weeks and involves warming the entire body for around 15 minutes one to three times a day for three to five days a week in an infrared sauna, after which the patient rests under blankets for an additional 30 minutes. This is followed by drinking an amount of water that corresponds to body weight lost through perspiration.

Saunas generally stimulate sweating, which can increase detoxification. However, every sweat gland has a sympathetic nerve attached to it and FIR for long COVID should be done gently and for only around 10 to 15 minutes maximum at a time, giving you the benefit of FIR without sweating profusely and so reduce the possibility that you will overstimulate the sympathetic nerves and aggravate your symptoms.

Antidepressants

When one is very poorly with any protracted illness, there is a recovery mountain to climb in order to get better. When one embarks on any treatment programme and symptoms start to improve, it is akin to climbing a mountain. As patients get higher and higher, they look down and feel sad and depressed that they were so ill. When they look up, their anxiety increases as they realise how much further they have to go until they reach 'the summit'. So, patients' moods will often change as they improve. It was noticeable in the clinical trials that we carried out at Salford University in the 1990s that, as the treated patients' fatigue, pain and cognitive function improved, their anxiety and depression scores dipped in the middle of the year-long trial, but picked up again when the summit became closer and the patients showed further improvement, helping reduce the anxiety and depression in the long term. This, at least, showed that ME/CFS is not a psychological disorder in which the other symptoms would correspond to depression or anxiety scores. However, antidepressants are sometimes used in ME/CFS and long COVID treatment.

The COVID-19 pandemic has caused extensive job losses around the world, leading to some men in certain communities that still endorse an old-fashioned masculine ideology of being the provider for the family, becoming particularly sensitive to status loss and thereby becoming an increased risk for suicidality.[6]

In the aftermath to the main pandemic, there has also been an increase in neuropsychiatric symptoms in patients with long COVID. For years doctors wrongly classed ME/CFS as a primary depressive disorder and equally now long COVID has been shown to be associated with diagnoses of depression,[7] with some viewing it as more of a neuropsychiatric disorder leading to depression, anxiety, post-traumatic stress disorder and sleep disturbances.[8]

However, since toxins can affect any region of the brain when they build-up in the nervous system, the limbic system controlling the emotional side of the brain could easily be the main focus of neuro-inflammation.

The same could be happening with long COVID and I have witnessed many long COVID patients with different psychological disorders as a result of the illness. Some get so depressed that they have suicidal thoughts and in some tragic cases can't go on any more.

As Professor of Psychiatry Leo Sher of Icahn School of Medicine at Mount Sinai, New York, warns in his 2023 paper on long COVID and the risk of suicide:[9] 'Families of individuals with long COVID need to be educated that psychiatric symptoms, especially suicidal ideation in long COVID patients, should be taken seriously. It is necessary to advise families of long COVID patients to get immediate professional medical help if individuals with long COVID experience suicidal thoughts.'

Some patients definitely need more than just my treatment and advice, and some do need to seek psychological or even psychiatric help.

Low doses of tricyclic antidepressants are prescribed to long COVID patients as they have been shown to improve the sleep patterns of some ME/CFS sufferers.[10] However, some of the older generation of antidepressants are habit-forming and may result in significant physical and psychological side effects, while certain foods have to be avoided while taking some antidepressants as they can cause harmful reactions. There are fewer such problems with today's antidepressants. However, if you are prescribed medication that aggravates your symptoms, you should return to your doctor to discuss the option of an alternative antidepressant. This is the same for all pharmaceutical approaches to treatment, including herbal remedies. In other words, if a drug reduces one or more of the symptoms with no major side effect, it may prove helpful in the battle against long COVID. However, if the reaction to the medicine outweighs the overall benefit or if it worsens the symptoms, you should immediately consult your GP or specialist in order to review the alternatives.

One of the best natural antidepressants is the amino acid tryptophan which the body needs to produce serotonin. Tryptophan is contained in many foods such as nuts, seeds, tofu, cheese, red meat, poultry, fish, oats, beans, lentils, and eggs. One can also take a much stronger dose of tryptophan in the form of 5HTP which you can buy over the counter without a prescription.

Another natural antidepressant is the plant St John's wort (*Hypericum perforatum*), sometimes sold as just 'Hypericum'. It contains the ingredients hypericin and hyperforin, which are used for their antidepressant properties. Both tryptophan and hypericum stimulate the release of the neurotransmitter serotonin, reducing depressing thoughts, and should be taken with your doctor's knowledge and, hopefully, guidance.

There are plenty of antidepressant medicines known as SSRIs ('selective serotonin reuptake inhibitors') which allow serotonin to stay in the brain for longer and so can help, but if one definitely needs to be prescribed antidepressants, I recommend patients ask their doctor for one in the group of SNRIs which should be taken in the morning. This group includes duloxetine, which has helped some of my patients by inhibiting the reuptake of noradrenalin (norepinephrine) as well as serotonin, so it stimulates more brain activity. Since we now know that in health the hypothalamus–locus–coeruleus axis is switched off during delta-wave sleep at night to help drain the brain of toxins, it makes sense to stimulate noradrenalin production in the morning, not at night when we want a more 'relaxed' switched-off brain to help improve restorative delta-wave sleep.

Researchers at Penn State University, Philadelphia have identified that infections in the gut trigger an inflammatory response due to cytokines that impair the gut's ability to absorb tryptophan, leading to a reduction in circulating serotonin impairing cognitive function due to disturbed vagal nerve activity from the gut.[11]

The gut–brain axis is a two-way affair which allows the brain to exert a major influence on intestinal activities and as important is the influence of the gut on mood, cognition and mental health.

The intestinal microbiome influences brain chemistry and behaviour, independently producing the majority of neurotransmitters and over 90% of total serotonin. It therefore follows that for a healthy biochemistry in the brain you need a healthy gut with the good bacteria working well and, as explained previously (page 22), gut dysbiosis is very common in long COVID affecting the gut–brain axis. So, besides any antidepressants the gut should be looked into and treated if necessary to help any depression or anxiety in the patient. Nutritional advice is given further on in this chapter.[12]

Acceptance and commitment therapy (ACT)

ACT is based on concepts and values of mindfulness and was developed by American psychologist Steven C Hayes PhD, who explained in an online interview: 'When I developed an anxiety disorder around 1980, I found that my behavioral and cognitive training failed me. I turned to my eastern roots, and also explored the human potential movement. That gave me a route forward personally and I eventually integrated all of that into the intellectual and practical work that became ACT.'[13]

Using ACT, the patient accepts and makes room for any challenges life may throw at them rather than fight them, while practising mindfulness, distress tolerance and emotion regulation. In CBT, patients are trained to challenge distressing thoughts. In ACT, the thought is accepted as a thought and then defused using a variety of techniques.

As already explained, if the main cause of neuro-inflammation is emotional stress, ACT helps the person be present in the moment and learn to accept painful or stressful thoughts and emotions. It is a useful tool for many people struggling with mood, thought, anxiety or personality disorders, but it has also been shown to help reduce chronic pain.[14]

In chronic pain, the main brain activity promoting the pain has been shown to shift from the standard neural pathway seen in acute pain to the areas in the brain more involved with the emotions. In other words, in acute pain, receptors around the body known as nociceptors send messages up the spine to the pain centres in the brain, including the thalamus. The nociceptors seem to have much less influence on chronic pain, which is experienced due to areas in the brain such as the amygdala being very active.

ACT trains the person to notice an uncomfortable emotion or thought and acknowledge it, but to let it flow by, without holding on to it or letting it drive actions in that moment. So, when one has chronic pain, the best thing to do is not to try to fight it head on or to simply ignore it. To reduce the pain, accept it and focus on any other goals you have now and let the pain flow by. It is difficult for severely ill, bedridden patients to have any goals to focus on other than their illness, but the meditation and mindfulness aspect of ACT has helped many people escape from a life of misery with unending pain.[15, 16, 17]

I have been asked by some patients over the years how I have managed to keep cheerful and positive when facing many stressful and challenging periods of my life. I use a similar approach to ACT. I call it the 'Perrin Woosh'. I let stressful events pass me by going 'Woosh!' right over my head, not stopping to make their mark but not ignoring them either. It might look as though I don't care, but it isn't that at all. I just focus on the things that are going in the right direction and accept the things I cannot change at the time and let them 'Woosh' by, away from any immediate harm to yours truly.

Another strategy I employ is what I term 'optimistic pessimism'. If things are not going right in my life, I imagine the very worst-case scenario. It might seem a crazy way of coping, but when the very worst doesn't happen – and invariably it doesn't – I am happy. This is similar to negative visualisation practised in ancient time by the Stoics, who visualised misfortunes long in advance, which they then felt better prepared for and ultimately led to greater tranquility.

It reminds me of a famous quotation from the legendary American actor and comedian, George Burns, who lived to be 100. When he reached his 90th birthday he was asked by a journalist, 'Mr Burns, how does it feel to be 90?' He dutifully replied: 'Well, I'll tell you. I get up every morning and read the obituary column. If my name's not there I eat breakfast.'

Warning: There are many forms of talking therapy available but, as I emphasise again and again in this book, patients also require a physical approach for a physical illness. Words alone via the psychological approach may reduce stress and help patients cope better but will not rid them of long COVID. Patients should be aware that some talking therapists may encourage them to do far too much too soon, or worse, lay the blame on them, the patient, if the approach doesn't work. Patients should never blame themselves or force themselves to increase activity because they have been told that this is the best way forward.

Acupuncture

Some long COVID patients suffer from severe pain in all parts of their bodies, similar to fibromyalgia patients. Some patients with fibromyalgia have benefited from acupuncture, the ancient Chinese form of medicine, which can be done as an adjunct to the Perrin Technique™. By inserting fine needles under the skin, western medical acupuncture stimulates the body's natural endorphins that reduce pain and promote healing.

A course of acupuncture can lead to longer lasting pain relief, often after a single treatment. Traditional acupuncture is based on the belief that a 'life force' or qi (pronounced 'chee') flows along pathways of the body known as meridians. The ancient Chinese belief is that stagnation of qi leads to disease and that acupuncture can re-establish the flow of this energy and restore health. Perhaps the qi in some way is related to lymphatic drainage which, when stagnated, or flowing the wrong way, leads to diseases such as long COVID? Food for thought …

Myofascial trigger-point dry-needling

Fascia is the connective tissue, primarily formed of collagen, found beneath the skin and that attaches, encloses and separates muscles plus other internal organs. The myofascial tissue is the fascia that is attached to the muscles and contains a rich network of lymphatic vessels. In long COVID, the myofascial layers may be too tight and cause much of the superficial pain.

Myofascial trigger-point dry-needling, simply known by many as dry-needling or intramuscular stimulation (IMS), is similar to acupuncture as it uses needles on certain myofascial trigger points which are specific tender points that can become tight and often painful when there is mechanical disturbance in the area. Dry-needling can treat a dysfunction of skeletal muscle and connective tissue, minimise pain and improve or regulate structural or functional damage.

Ozone therapy

We often hear on the news that the ozone layer in the atmosphere, which protects us from the sun's harmful rays, is being affected by planetary pollution. Ozone is formed naturally following lightning in thunderstorms and is actually a molecule of the oxygen we breathe (O_2) with an extra oxygen atom attached (O_3). It is a formidable steriliser and a powerful antimicrobial agent. The extra atom of oxygen creates a reactive form of the gas and, via the process known as oxidation, destroys the walls of bacteria and viruses and afterwards reverts back to the harmless oxygen that we breathe.

Ozone therapy can be useful in treating inflamed and painful tissue by targeting and destroying the cells responsible for the damage.

Some patients who have connective tissue and hypermobility disorders, such as Ehlers-Danlos syndrome, have been helped using a treatment known as prolozone therapy. Prolozone therapy uses injections of nutrients to increase the amount of collagen and cartilage in a weak or damaged region of the body, thereby regenerating new tissue together with ozone to destroy the damaged ligaments. The action of prolozone therapy helps strengthen hypermobile painful joints. By repairing the damaged tissue, it can reduce the chronic pain that causes misery to long COVID patients, as it has helped with ME/CFS and FMS.[18]

Earthing

Earthing is based on the fact that the Earth's surface contains an endless number of electrons, and its negative potential can help the neutralisation of free radicals in the body, similar to the action of antioxidants (page 171), helping restore balanced health. It has been scientifically shown that, by walking barefoot on the outside ground and using specially produced conductive products, such as earthing mats, a more harmonious balance is achieved in the electromagnetic fields within the organs that can improve health. Fluctuation in the strength of the Earth's potential may also help regulate a person's biological clock. Coming into contact with the Earth also energises the body plus aids the regulation of the autonomic nervous system, reducing the sympathetic overload seen in disease processes. This could aid neuro-lymphatic drainage and reduce many of the symptoms in long COVID.

Colonic irrigation (colonic hydrotherapy)

Colonic irrigation is a form of hydrotherapy that involves flushing waste material out of the bowel using water (sometimes containing herbal preparations) and is often more effective than using an enema. It should always be carried out by a trained practitioner and under the guidance of your doctor, as there are some known side effects, such as anaemia, and it is not recommended for inflammatory bowel disorders and some other serious diseases. Of course, one has to replace the healthy gut bacteria removed in the process and so probiotics are required after the colon has been irrigated. By cleansing out toxins stuck in the bowel this method could prove useful for some long COVID patients and has been shown to help symptoms of irritable bowel syndrome, such as pain, constipation and diarrhoea.[19]

Vagal nerve stimulation

As discussed earlier in the book, the vagus nerve, the main nerve of the parasympathetic nervous system, if stimulated can help reduce cytokine activity and therefore help with the neuro-inflammation found in long COVID.[20, 21]

Heart rate variability (HRV), which is used as a measure of autonomic control, is increased when the vagus nerve is stimulated together with reducing the neuro-inflammation thus improving health in many conditions.

Therefore, scientists have used vagal nerve stimulation to help patients with long COVID with some success.[22]

- A transcutaneous vagal nerve stimulator has been shown to provide improvements on a few biomarkers of cognition and mood.
- In a study by Thakkar and colleagues there was a significant benefit of a transcutaneous vagal nerve stimulator neuromodulation compared to placebo across all test questions in a range of cognitive tests examining memory.[23]
- A transcutaneous vagal nerve stimulator significantly improved speed on learning tasks compared with controls.[24]

However, some patients have an irritation of their dorsal vagus (as discussed in Chapters 1 and 4) and, if this is exacerbated by a vagal nerve stimulator, it could lead to pathological mechanisms that cause symptoms such as extremely slow heart rate and sleep apnoea, so, as with all treatments for long COVID, go gently and stop immediately if symptoms worsen.

Immunological therapies

An alternative term for ME/CFS in the USA used to be chronic fatigue and immune dysfunction syndrome (CFIDS), an acknowledgement that dysfunction of the immune system is a major feature of the disease, as is the case with long COVID. However, many immune modulatory treatments are expensive and not freely available, produce unpleasant side effects and yield inconclusive results.

Many antiviral and antibiotic therapies have also been tried for ME/CFS over the past 50 years, especially when the patient has a history of persistent or long-term infections such as the Epstein-Barr virus that initiates glandular fever, also known as infectious mononucleosis or 'mono'.

Over the years, I have stressed that although there may be some viral or other infections that preceded the onset of the major symptoms, when you look back at the history of the patient (or yourself if you are the patient!) you inevitably find many difficulties in their health, and earlier symptoms that eventually built up over the years until triggered by an event, which is usually a viral infection, that leads to ME/CFS. In long COVID this trigger is obviously the SARS-CoV-2 virus. In other words, I believe the problem is pre-viral and the COVID-19 infection is the final trigger of the disease and never the singular cause. After all, billions of people worldwide have been infected with the coronavirus and, although they may have been unwell for weeks after, they have fully recovered. So, what prevents long COVID patients from recovering like most other people?

The clue is in one of the names given to ME/CFS – that is, 'post-viral' or 'post-infectious fatigue'. After the invading organism has infected the body, the immune system sends out large protein signalling cytokines to activate immune cells to destroy the virus These cytokines then require removal via lymphatic drainage. This process we know is compromised and reversed in long COVID, as discussed extensively throughout this book.

Apheresis, plasmapheresis (TPE) and immunoadsorption

Apheresis is a process developed in 1972 where blood is passed through a machine that separates out one particular constituent and returns the remainder to the circulation. Plasma, the fluid part of the blood, is a light-yellow liquid composed of water, salts and enzymes which helps in the removal of waste from the body as well as carrying all parts of the blood through the circulatory system.

Plasmapheresis, also known as 'therapeutic plasma exchange' (TPE), is the removal of plasma from the patient and separation by a machine into component parts, some of which are returned to the patient. This procedure may be effective in some cases of long COVID when regulation of the immune response is disturbed and auto-antibodies are present, as shown in some other serious illnesses.[25]

One should be cautious before beginning with this technique as during plasma exchange, blood pressure is lowered and so the technique is not suitable for patients who already have lowered blood pressure. Drinking lots of water in the days before treatment can reduce common reactions such as nausea and dizziness. Some patients have suffered from bleeds and other allergic reactions following plasmapheresis.

Immunoadsorption (IA-treatment) is another method that may help long COVID patients; it uses a different type of machine to remove specific antibodies from the blood without the need for TPE. In a study on 178 patients diagnosed with post-COVID syndrome, Giszas and colleagues discovered raised AAb-levels (anti-ß1/ß2 and anti-M3/M4 receptors). The authors describe the clinical courses of two patients with elevated AAb-levels that underwent IA-treatment, achieving short-term reductions in AAb-levels and symptom remission in one of the two patients who was treated with IA, but who relapsed to a worse state after six weeks, so much further research needs to be implemented on this novel approach.[26]

Low-dose naltrexone (LDN)

Another medical approach that has been shown to help some patients with their symptoms is low-dose naltrexone (LDN) which is the 'off-label' use of the medication naltrexone at low doses for diseases such as multiple sclerosis and fibromyalgia.[27, 28] Naltrexone is typically prescribed for opioid or alcohol dependence, as it is a strong opioid antagonist. Opioid receptors modulate pain reception in the body and also increase the production of the body's natural endorphins. They have also been shown to be important in the immune system by regulating cell proliferation in certain cells, such as T and B lymphocytes and tumour cells.[29]

The reason LDN may also help is that it may act as an anti-inflammatory agent in the central nervous system, especially on the glia,[30] which contain many pro-inflammatory cytokines and other neurotoxins that build up in long COVID.

Conclusion

As shown in this chapter there are other emerging treatments for long COVID that help some, but as I stated in Chapter 6, there is no magic bullet for long COVID as it is not the type of disease where there can be a one size fits all approach. The key to treating any complex disorders is by finding a treatment that helps and then another that helps and building up a multidisciplinary approach, tailor-made for each individual patient.

Professor David Putrino, the director of rehabilitation innovation for Mount Sinai Health System based in New York, gave a wonderful lecture to a conference I attended at New York State University, Stonybrook in 2023,[31] where he likened the problem of treating complex disorders such as long COVID to a ship weighed down by multiple anchors. If one anchor is drawn up from the sea bed and the ship doesn't move then you don't drop that anchor back in the water and try and haul up the next one. You have to keep all anchors raised before the ship can move. This analogy best fits the treatment of most of the long COVID patients I have so far treated in clinic.

The therapies mentioned in this chapter may help. However, incorporating the Perrin Technique™ in the early intervention of all long COVID patients may help and indeed prevent, to some significant degree, the emergence of post-viral symptoms that are resistant to the treatments described above.

As my colleagues and I suggested to the medical world in our preliminary report in 2022,[32] the addition of the Perrin Technique™ could enhance the multidisciplinary approach established by Halpin and colleagues[33] in the UK to treat the post-viral fatigue-related states, alleviate symptoms and improve the quality of life of those millions affected by long COVID.

Chapter 9

Diet and supplements

'What did they live on?' said Alice, who always took a great interest in questions of eating and drinking.

'They lived on treacle' said the Dormouse, after thinking a minute or two.

'They couldn't have done that, you know,' Alice gently remarked; 'they'd have been ill.'

'So they were' said the Dormouse; 'very ill.'

Lewis Carroll

Alice's Adventures in Wonderland

Janine's story

I am a 60-year-old woman, married with adult children, who had worked since university as a lawyer in private practice, until becoming unwell. I had a very busy life and was generally fit and healthy until five years ago when I was diagnosed first with severe depression. Second, in short order, in March 2020 I got COVID-19, right at the start of the pandemic. I was extremely ill, initially developing a fever coupled with what felt like an electric shock/

extreme burning sensation running through my body in waves. This burning sensation peaked at night so I was unable to sleep. Contrary to most COVID-19 cases, I had no initial respiratory symptoms other than a severe sore throat, although I was from the outset extremely fatigued. I had a very painful right elbow joint and have continued to experience palpitations and pain in my right lower abdomen.

The fever resolved after a week, but the other symptoms did not improve. I spent the following three weeks hardly out of bed and each night the symptoms started to peak in the evening. I was getting no sleep and was exhausted. After a month I was referred to the neurological team and prescribed both pain relief and sleeping tablets. The diagnosis was that I had peripheral nerve damage from the viral infection, which would hopefully resolve over the next year or so. It seemed that the virus had attacked my nervous system in particular, potentially because that was a weak area for me.

I struggled on, managing to do limited household tasks but otherwise living a very restricted life due to both chronic fatigue and continuing depression. A friend then recommended the Perrin Clinic to me in the summer of 2020, and I first saw Raymond Perrin in August 2020. At an initial consultation, I was diagnosed with post-COVID/post-viral fatigue syndrome. I believe that other factors were stress and restricted spinal movement. Both these factors made sense to me, as my work had become extremely stressful, and I had suffered with back pain for years.

I began attending weekly sessions with Raymond and his osteopathic colleague Antoinette, which I continued for the first year, and then every two weeks, and still attend regular appointments. I am not yet at the point where I am able to live and work as before, as I have to manage my level of activity – otherwise I find my symptoms become more intense and debilitating. However, I am very much improved, and I am hopeful that this will continue with regular treatment.

Janine Allen, Bury, Greater Manchester.
Patient of Dr Perrin and licensed Perrin Technique™ practitioner
Antionette Atuah

Diet and nutrition

I have learnt, over the years that no one diet is the universal answer for neuro-lymphatic disorders. Some patients with long COVID respond badly to some diets; other patients swear by particular regimes. The main rule is that any specific dietary plans should always be followed under the supervision of a trained health professional who can assess what is right for the individual patient without the risk of nutritional deficiencies.

As a general rule I would advise all patients to eat regular, healthy meals and drink plenty of healthy fluids, such as filtered or bottled mineral water – 2 litres a day for an adult should be enough.

Irritable bowel syndrome (IBS) and gut dysbiosis

One of the common symptoms of long COVID is irritable bowel syndrome (IBS) which takes the form (usually) of loose bowels and/or constipation, bloating and pain in any part of the abdomen. This is in part due to the dysfunction of the sympathetic nerves controlling the smooth muscles of the bowel wall. The irritable bowel in long COVID usually occurs together with gut dysbiosis.

Gut dysbiosis is the term used for an imbalance in the flora in the gut, the gut 'microbiota', with normally dominant healthy bacteria overtaken by harmful bacteria, viruses and fungi, including candida. The beneficial microbial colonies aid healthy digestion and also help protect the body from pathogens. These benefits are lost when the balance tips in favour of harmful micro-organisms.

The way the cells in our body react to disease relies on what is known as the 'gene expression' of a cell. As many scientists keep on saying, 'it's all in the genes'. We now know that the expression of genes can change and often does due to external influence, such as increased toxins. This is known as 'epigenetics'.

The genes of all the microbes in our bodies are known collectively as the 'human microbiome'. There are 10 times more bacterial cells than human cells in any human body and these bacterial cells contain five to eight million genes compared with ours, which number about 20,000. A healthy diet is required to improve the health of all the microbiome to fight disease, especially in conditions that affect the whole body, such as long COVID. So, in theory, viruses and bacteria can lead to many intolerances and switch on genes that wrongly cause our body to recognise regular foods as harmful, leading to autoimmune reactions and disorders, such as coeliac disease.

Microbial colonies excrete waste by-products and the excess waste, especially larger molecules, require a healthy lymphatic system to process them. When there is also a leaky gut as a result of damage to the gut lining from harmful microbes, these waste products, plus yeast, gluten and the milk protein casein (which are all large molecules and need to drain via the lymphatics), will overburden the lymphatic system, which, if the person has long COVID, will additionally be pumping the lymph in the wrong direction.

For this reason, sugar, wheat and other gluten-based foods plus dairy products should be reduced in long COVID, especially if the patient suffers from IBS.

Do specific diets help?

The FODMAP diet

One of the key approaches to reducing the symptoms of this functional disorder is known as the FODMAP diet. 'FODMAP' stands for a group of poorly-absorbed sugars found in some fruit and vegetables, milk and wheat – namely, **F**ermentable, **O**ligosaccharides, **D**isaccharides, **M**onosaccharides **A**nd **P**olyols. High FODMAP foods include, for example, common dietary items like apples, milk, broccoli, leeks, garlic, onions, peas, dried beans, bread, breakfast cereals, biscuits, barley, beer and fruit juices.

The process of drawing fluid into the bowel and the fermentation of FODMAPs by bacteria has been identified as one of the causes of the symptoms experienced by people with IBS. Reducing the intake of high-FODMAP foods can help reduce symptoms of IBS.

However, not all FODMAP foods may be bad for the individual and anyone eliminating FODMAPs should try to reintroduce some after a four-to-eight-week restriction diet. It has been shown that some FODMAPs have pre-biotic qualities that are important in maintaining the good bacteria in the gut, so it isn't a good idea to go on a total FODMAP exclusion diet for too long.

Other special diets

Some patients swear by regimes such as the paleolithic (paleo) diet (also known as the Stone Age diet) which is made up of foods that in ancient times were obtained by hunting and gathering rather than the farming methods of the last few thousand years. A paleo diet therefore includes foods such as meat, fish, fruit, vegetables, nuts and seeds but no dairy, grains or processed foods.

Others find they are helped by the ketogenic diet which is low-carb, high-fibre and high-fat, and has been shown in clinical trials to help reverse type 2 diabetes and reduce epilepsy symptoms. There are, however, reasons why a high-fat diet may be problematic in long COVID. The lymphatic fluid around the bowel, which is known as chyle, absorbs fat and is thus creamy white in colour, unlike the clear, colourless lymphatic fluid in the rest of the body. Excess fat in the diet may worsen the situation when there is a reversal of normal lymphatic flow. The fat may not drain away in the chyle but may remain congested in the gut. This resultant build-up of fat becomes a collecting depot for further neurotoxins.

Some practitioners and their patients combine these two diets, as in the paleo-ketogenic (PK) diet advocated by independent naturopathic doctor, Dr Sarah Myhill among others, for its benefits in counteracting 'the upper fermenting gut' and being the best support for the mitochondria (see page 239).[1] It is, however, a difficult diet to follow for vegans/plant-based eaters whose main source of protein will be legumes, which are relatively high in carbohydrates.

On the opposite end of the nutritional spectrum, plant-based diets have been shown to help many symptoms of long COVID, including fatigue, sleep disorders, headaches, mood swings and pain and are advocated by some nutritionists.[2]

It is always a case of trial and error until you find what best suits you.

Exclusion diets

Some of the weakest, most emaciated and immobile patients I have seen are those who have been following strict avoidance diets, often for many years. They usually start by being slightly intolerant of certain foods and, within some months of avoiding those, may become completely intolerant of many. As time goes on, more intolerances seem to develop, with the body's immune system going into 'free fall' mode, and the patient rapidly descending into a state where nearly every food, perfume or deodorant causes adverse reactions, as seen in mast cell activation syndrome (see page 21) becoming more and more prevalent in long COVID patients.

So, my advice is that in the early stages, if any food sensitivity has been discovered, do not abstain totally for more than a month and, occasionally cheat, eating a little of that substance. The exception to this rule would be if the patient was proved to be allergic, as with peanut allergy for example, or to have coeliac disease when one cannot tolerate any gluten at all.

Processed and ultra-processed foods: An exception to this rule not to abstain totally relates to processed foods. These should be avoided as much as possible and brown flour and brown sugar should replace the white varieties. Ultra-processed foods (UPFs) should be completely avoided. These are not just the foods bought in fast-food outlets, such as takeaway fried chicken or snacks such as artificially-flavoured tortilla chips and fruit-drinks with artificial colours and flavourings, but many products on supermarket shelves that you would think of as reasonably healthy, like oat cereal with added chocolate. Numerous studies have shown that diets high in ultra-processed foods lead to many diseases, including cancer, diabetes and dementia. In a recent study in the UK examining the risk of cancer and associated death rates linked to UPFs, the mean UPF consumption was shown to be a staggering 22.9% of the total diet, leading to the conclusion that a higher UPF intake may be linked to an increase in cancer with higher mortality rates.[3]

Smoking: This is of course not part of nutrition/diet but this seems a good place to emphasise that I am also totally against smoking as it has so many proven detrimental effects on health; however, the stress of trying to stop smoking may be too much for some patients and place excess strain on the sympathetic nervous system so, as much as I hate saying this, for some patients who haven't any respiratory symptoms, it may be better to continue smoking than attempting to quit while they are trying to recover from long COVID.

Drinks

As I've said above, patients should drink plenty of healthy fluids, such as filtered or bottled mineral water – 2 litres a day for an adult should be enough.

Stimulants such as caffeine are to be reduced and avoided altogether if possible. Caffeine takes a very long time for its stimulatory effects to wear off so patients should avoid any caffeine in the afternoon and evening. Decaffeinated coffee and decaffeinated tea can be drunk instead although most still contain some caffeine and decaffeinated coffee has been shown to increase cholesterol levels, so this should be taken only in moderation. Herbal teas or naturally caffeine-free teas such as Rooibos/Red Bush are preferable.

Alcohol

Alcohol is an absolute no-no for anyone with long COVID. This is for two fundamental reasons – alcohol damages the liver which is essential for detoxing, and it has disastrous effects on the brain.

The detrimental effects alcohol has on the liver are well documented and it is known that alcohol is the main cause of cirrhosis and liver disease. The main aim of the Perrin Technique™ is to drain toxins out of the central nervous system into the lymphatic system. The lymphatics will eventually drain the toxins into the bloodstream, with most ending up in the liver, which will need support rather than an extra further toxic load provided by alcohol.

However, the main reason why even a small amount of alcohol aggravates long COVID, is due to its effect on key areas of the brain that are disrupted by a backflow of the neuro-lymphatics into the brain. As discussed earlier, research has shown that when the drainage of lymphatic fluid through the perivascular spaces is stopped there is a build-up of toxins in the thalamus and basal ganglia of the brain. The thalamus contains high levels of N-methyl-D-aspartate (NMDA). The methyl in the name is the clue, as this is the neurochemical affected when one drinks any alcohol and it is this neurotransmitter, as well as GABA in the basal ganglia, that causes many of the symptoms of drunkenness. In long COVID, NMDA overstimulation leads to increased pain and more sleep disturbance as well as reduced cognitive function. So, alcohol, even a tiny drop, will usually worsen a patient's symptoms and, indeed, many patients find they cannot tolerate much alcohol anyway, with a small amount making them feel drunk.

Neurologist Georgia Lea MD posted an article entitled 'Could a glass of wine diagnose long COVID?' in March 2021.[4] She wrote: 'Before getting COVID, I routinely had a beer or glass of wine at dinner but starting with my first beer during quarantine (I was alone with our beer fridge!) I couldn't tolerate more than 2 to 3 sips. Yes, you read that correctly. By the second or third sip of alcohol, I feel a not-so-great "buzz" of light-headedness, sluggishness, and queasiness'.

This is also why I advise patients to try to have vaccines that have been preserved by freezing and so have no alcohol in their content. The last thing a long COVID patient needs is a direct injection of alcohol into the bloodstream, even a minute amount.

In the case of COVID vaccines, however, those that were frozen (produced by Pfizer) were the mRNA vaccines which carried a piece of spike protein that could travel into the brain of many people with prior disturbed neuro-lymphatic system. As mentioned on page 26 in the stages leading to long COVID, stage 5 includes the spike protein of the COVID-19 virus entering the brain and leading to neuro-inflammation. So, if we introduce a spike protein into the body and the lymphatic system is already working in reversal it doesn't take a brain surgeon to work out what might happen next.

So, in the early days of vaccines patients had a dilemma – do I take alcohol or a spike protein into my body? The proverbial 'Catch 22'. Unfortunately, I didn't have any crystal ball but since the other vaccines at the time seemed to contain more chemicals that could affect my ME/CFS patients, including the alcohol, I advised if patients chose to have the vaccine, then they should receive the mRNA vaccine if a choice was possible. I actually received the AstraZeneca vaccine for the first two jabs as my vaccine centre didn't give me the choice and I didn't have ME/CFS. Both vaccines did have side effects and some people across the world have suffered from severe reactions from mRNA vaccines.[5]

However, my advice to my patients was possibly vindicated by a report from the NHS Business Services in 2023, which operates the vaccine damage scheme. The report showed less frequent severe adverse reactions with the mRNA vaccines and revealed that by 6 March 2023, of the claims relating to a COVID-19 vaccine that had been processed, 622 concerned the AstraZeneca vaccine, 348 the Pfizer, and 43 the Moderna vaccine.[6]

Tinctures

Before I leave the subject of alcohol and move on to the more positive topic of nutritional supplements, I need to include a note about tinctures. Many supplements come in the form of tinctures in little bottles which allow droplets of the remedy to be taken easily into the body rather than in pill or capsule form. The liquid medium of the tincture is usually alcohol-based and so, if one takes tinctures of supplements containing alcohol, then drop them into hot water first which will evaporate the alcohol, then wait until the water has cooled down before drinking the safe mixture.

Supplements – an overview

As well as a healthy diet, a supplement of vitamins C, D and B complex is advised. The former increases the patient's general resistance to infection, D maintains respiratory health and aids modulation of the immune response, while B complex improves energy production and general functioning of the nervous system. As mentioned in Chapter 6, I recommend a daily dose for adults of 500 mg vitamin C, 600–2000 IU (international units) vitamin D, especially in regions of the world with dark winter days where less natural vitamin D is synthesised by sunlight, plus a strong, or whole, B complex tablets are recommended.

Vitamins B and C are both water-soluble so that excess is excreted from the body, as long as it is not too large an amount. However, one of the functions of vitamin C is to aid the absorption of calcium, so there is a risk of developing kidney stones if the vitamin C intake is too high. I always try to err to the side of caution and so this is why I advise patients to take only 500 mg a day. Vitamin D is fat soluble, so it is important not to overload the system, especially as the lymphatics are involved in the transport of fat-soluble vitamins such as vitamin D.

Beware of taking so many different supplements that any possible benefit is likely to be outweighed by undesired side effects. In addition, many supplements can have an adverse reaction with other medications and may exert a strain on the gut as well as the liver and thus the lymphatics and the sympathetic nervous system. This will undoubtedly worsen the symptoms of long COVID, as I have seen in some long COVID patients I am treating at present in clinic.

One of my ME/CFS patients years ago was taking so many supplements and prescribed medications that the first instruction I gave to her was to reduce all these supplements and go back to her doctor and check which medications she could stop or reduce the dose of (see Fig. 44). It took quite a while for her body to pick up after reducing this overload of supplementation and medication. However, together with the treatment she received from myself and one of my colleagues, she began to recover as is clearly demonstrated in the photo of her taken a few years on (see Fig. 45). It is always best to seek expert professional advice when taking any medicinal treatments, whether pharmaceutical or herbal. So, speak to your doctor, pharmacist, naturopath, nutritionist or herbalist to find out what is best for you.

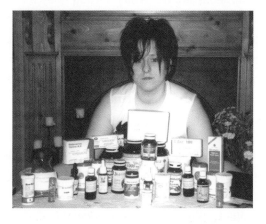

Fig. 44 An ME/CFS patient and her daily medications.

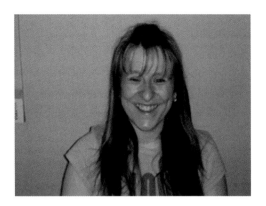

Fig. 45 The same patient after receiving the Perrin Technique™ and reducing her supplements and medication intake.

Even though excessive use is harmful, there are times when supplements may be necessary.

Vitamin and mineral supplements

Kazimierz Funk (1884–1967), a Polish biochemist, is generally credited with being among the first to formulate (in 1912) the concept of vitamins. The word 'vitamin' is formed from the words 'vital' and 'amine' and indicates that these chemical compounds are necessary for the body's metabolism to work properly. They are usually inadequately produced by the body and therefore extra must be included in our diet or taken as a supplement. Vitamins are widely recommended in the treatment of long COVID. The Association of UK Dietitians (the BDA) in January 2022 advised patients should be given a balanced diet with a wide variety of vitamins, minerals, protein, energy, fibre and fluid to work best and help recovery.

The antioxidant action of vitamin C has been shown to improve the body's immune response. With patients taking no more than 500 mg per day, there have been no reported toxic side-effects. Similarly, the vitamin B group is known to improve the health of the nervous system.

Some doctors specialising in neuro-immune conditions give high doses of vitamin C and folic acid intravenously which is safe if closely monitored by the prescribing physician. I, however, err on the side of caution and advise a 500 mg daily oral supplement of vitamin C and one complete vitamin B-complex pill to increase the patient's resistance to overall infection and improve cell energy production and the functioning of the nervous system.

Supplements and the mitochondria

Since one of the main symptoms of long COVID is a lack of energy, it follows that many researchers have looked at the energy production in the body as a possible explanation of the disease. The powerhouses of our cells (and those of all other animals) are known as the mitochondria and it is in these organelles that a major cycle of different reactions take place, the Krebs cycle, which is an essential biochemical pathway that our cells use to produce energy. To provide the key cofactors required for optimal energy output, we also need good methylation. The building blocks of proteins are known as amino acids. Specific amino acids are needed to produce different proteins, such as the neurotransmitters that send messages from one nerve to another, as has been discussed throughout this book. Different neurotransmitters are produced by slight differences to the amino acids, usually by the addition of a methyl group onto the existing amino acid; this is the process known as methylation. A methyl group consists of one carbon atom attached to three hydrogen atoms and is derived from the methane molecule with one hydrogen atom missing.

Methylation is a vital metabolic process that takes place in every cell in our body, occurring more than a billion times per second throughout the body. It is not only important for energy production but vital for the body's genetics, immunity, detoxification and brain function. The reactions that occur when one molecule passes a methyl group to another molecule produce chemicals vital for healthy energy metabolism, such as creatine, L carnitine, coenzyme Q10 (CoQ10) and homocysteine, which ultimately leads to the production of glutathione. These chemicals produced in the methylation cycle help power the Krebs cycle mentioned above, also known as the citric acid cycle (CAC) or the tricarboxylic acid (TCA) cycle. The Krebs cycle consists of a a series of chemical reactions to release stored energy through the oxidation of acetyl-coenzyme A, derived from carbohydrates, fats and proteins, into carbon dioxide and chemical energy by a process that ultimately converts the energy molecule adenosine triphosphate (ATP) into adenosine diphosphate (ADP) plus energy. As well as supporting energy production via the Krebs cycle, methylation is important for many other vital bodily functions, such as immune function, detoxification, balancing moods and reducing inflammation.

In my earlier days of attending international ME/CFS conferences there were a few characters at these events who stood out from the crowd. One such delegate was Rich van Konynenburg, a larger-than-life nuclear physicist, who formally proposed a biochemical model of stress-induced glutathione depletion in the disorder at a ME/ CFS Conference in Wisconsin in 2004.

Rich, who sadly died in 2012, maintained that glutathione, the master antioxidant in the body and a key player in the cellular energy production system, was depleted in the cells of ME/CFS patients, and he believed this leads to many of the dysfunctions found in ME/CFS.

In 2007 he re-engineered his theory and called it the 'glutathione depletion–methylation cycle block hypothesis' to incorporate his new understanding. He identified methylation as essential to produce vital molecules, such as CoQ-10 and L carnitine, and many others. It is also important in the production of myelin which forms electrically insulated sheaths around many nerves. He found it important in DNA expression and as part of folic acid metabolism, which also switches on synthesis of new DNA and RNA. The methylation cycle is also essential for cell-mediated immune function carried out by T lymphocytes and it requires many minerals and nutrients to work correctly, the main ones being magnesium and vitamin B12, which are often advised by naturopaths and nutritionists for long COVID as well as creatine, L carnitine, CoQ10, and glutathione.

In the body, CoQ10 (ubiquinone) is converted to the active form, ubiquinol, which is a more active compound, so I often recommend patients to take ubiquinol directly to improve their energy. In a clinical trial, CoQ10, also known as bio-quinine, has been shown to help reduce fatigue, help restore mitochondrial function and bioenergetic metabolism, and reduce oxidative stress in ME/CFS when taken together with a powerful form of vitamin B3, the coenzyme NADH. So, this combination should help many long COVID patients. Angela Bartletter and her colleagues in Italy showed that CoQ10 and the antioxidant alpha lipoic acid did just that.[7]

Supplements in detail

Magnesium supplementation

Magnesium deficiency, besides its effect on energy, is also associated with disorders of neuromuscular and psychiatric functioning and an inability to cope with viral infections.[8, 9] The two main forms of magnesium compound taken orally are magnesium maleate and magnesium citrate. In my experience it all depends on personal preference, but I usually advise magnesium maleate (or 'malate' in the US), which is a combination of the mineral magnesium and malic acid. Malic acid is a naturally occurring substance that aids energy production in the body. Some patients may find the citrate or other versions work better than maleate, and, as I keep emphasising, every patient is different and will find many different supplements that work best for them.

Patients with long COVID with severe widespread muscular pain as a major symptom resemble patients with fibromyalgia syndrome (FMS). They may find magnesium maleate the best option, as a study on fibromyalgia patients showed a possible difficulty in these patients in creating malic acid. A study of 24 people with FMS suggested that magnesium maleate taken for at least two months may relieve the pain and tenderness associated with the condition.[10] Magnesium citrate is preferred by some practitioners and is the product of magnesium combined with citric acid. Magnesium citrate is often used in liquid form as a saline laxative to treat constipation, or to completely empty the intestines prior to surgery, but it can be found in capsular form. There are some superior products with a combination of different forms of magnesium to account for the way different compounds are absorbed into the blood.

The problem with most magnesium supplements is that, while a product may have a label claiming to contain magnesium citrate, it may actually use magnesium oxide as a base to boost the label claim for the elemental amount of magnesium, and blend this with a carrier such as citrate. You need to ensure that the product contains *fully reacted* magnesium, which should be clearly stated on the label.

Magnesium oxide is both *inorganic* and *insoluble*, meaning that it is extremely poorly absorbed and simply passes through the gastrointestinal tract (often resulting in unpleasant laxative side effects). Patients should look for products that are fully reacted and which are directly bound to the carrier, with no magnesium oxide. Some products may be buffered, which combines fully reacted magnesium with magnesium oxide, but at least they are better than blends. A low dose of magnesium taken several times a day is better absorbed and retained.

One should seek medical advice before taking magnesium, especially if you have any kidney disorder. Magnesium can potentially interact with certain medications, including high blood pressure medicines and some antibiotics.

Chelation (the detoxification of heavy metals)

Magnesium maleate also has chelating properties in that it can bind to toxic heavy metals, such as lead and mercury or many lighter metals, such as aluminium, which are still highly neurotoxic and respond well to many chelation agents, reducing the toxic overload.[11]

Chlorella

As well as magnesium maleate, an excellent chelation agent that I recommend is *Chlorella pyrenoidosa*, a blue-green algae. Chlorella contains large amounts of vitamin K, a nutrient that helps the body's clotting function (but may interfere with blood-thinning effects of certain medications, such as warfarin and others). If you are severely immune compromised, or if you take immune-suppressive drugs, or if you have a heart condition, seek medical advice before taking chlorella supplements.

Coconut oil

Together with chlorella, I recommend taking 2 teaspoons of coconut oil per day. It can be added in cooking, used as a spread or eaten off the spoon. The coconut oil absorbs the chlorella and heavy metal combination.

One of the most important attributes of coconut oil is that it contains high levels of the family of fats known as medium-chain triglycerides (MCT) which are much smaller molecules than the long-chain triglycetrides (LCT). In the gut MCTs and LCTs are digested into their corresponding fatty acids. The LCTs form large lipoprotein molecules known as chylomicrons which turn the normally colourless lymph fluid into a creamy white solution known as chyle. Because of their size, the chylomicrons need the lymphatic system to drain away eventually into the blood via the thoracic duct whereas the small molecular MCTs do not require the lymphatic system. This means MCTs will not overload the lymphatic system in the gut as their shorter chains allow them to be absorbed directly into the blood capillaries and then go via the blood circulation to the liver where they are mostly oxidised for energy.[12]

However, some readers may question why taking the extra cholesterol found in coconut oil will help, given the long-running debate that too much cholesterol in the diet can lead to too much in the blood, which is associated with an increased risk of getting heart and circulatory diseases. This debate is not for this book, but it is worth noting that, while coconut oil is about 90% saturated fat, it also gives 'good' HDL cholesterol a boost in the following way.

Most of our cholesterol is made in the body by the liver. It is also found in many foods, including oils. It plays a vital part in how every cell works and is also needed to make vitamin D, some hormones and bile for digestion. Cholesterol is carried in the blood attached to proteins called lipoproteins. There are two main forms, LDL (low density lipoprotein), the 'bad, unhealthy cholesterol' and HDL (high density lipoprotein) the 'good, protective cholesterol'. Coconut oil contains healthy oils that are high in natural saturated fats which increase the healthy HDL cholesterol in your body.

Saturated fat is divided into various types, based on the number of carbon atoms in the molecule, and about half of the saturated fat in coconut oil is the 12-carbon variety, called lauric acid. That is a higher percentage than in most other oils and is probably responsible for its unusual HDL effects. However, plant-based oils are more than just fats. They contain many antioxidants and other substances which help long COVID patients.

Psyllium husks

Psyllium, or ispaghula, is the common name used for several members of the plant genus Plantago. Psyllium is mainly used as a dietary fibre to relieve symptoms of both constipation and mild diarrhoea and occasionally as a food thickener, and is totally gluten free, which is important. Taking a supplement of psyllium husks acts as roughage that helps with the removal and passage of the coconut oil, chlorella and heavy metal mix out through the alimentary canal. In some cases, one has to be careful about using psyllium, as it has been known sometimes to clog up the bowel. Basically, one should take the psyllium for the first month to 'get things moving' and avoid it completely if prone to constipation.

Activated charcoal

The ingestion of charcoal has also been used for centuries to help remove toxins from the body. Activated charcoal is produced at much higher temperatures than standard charcoal and is much more porous. Therefore, it is more effective in filtering impurities than standard charcoal. Takesumi, or carbonised bamboo, has been shown to be very helpful in the detoxification of many poisons, including food additives, heavy metals and other biotoxins that are found within the body. It does also have some antifungal and antibacterial properties.[13]

Vitamin B12

Vitamin B12 is useful with magnesium, as mentioned before, and there is evidence for its benefits combined with B9.[14] However, how the magnesium and vitamin B12 are administered depends on each individual practitioner and differs from case to case. Vitamin B12 injections, usually into the thigh or upper arm, in the form of either cyanocobalamin or hydroxocobalamin are probably the most efficient way of increasing your vitamin B12 levels.

A diet that includes meat, fish, eggs and dairy products can provide natural sources of B12 in the form of hydroxocobalamin, which is why B12 deficiency is very common in vegans. However, in numerous long COVID sufferers there is a problem in the disgestion of the vitamin in the stomach and its absorption in the small intestine, so many cannot rely on diet alone.

Symptoms of vitamin B12 deficiency include depression and mood disorders, fatigue, memory failure, anaemia, low blood pressure and nerve damage in the hands and feet. Follow the advice from your doctor as each case is different and some patients may be severely deficient and others may not have a problem at all, which is again another complexity of long COVID in that nutritionally no two patients require the same supplementation, and all dietary needs are different. Be aware, however, that B12 blood levels can be misleading as haematologists now recognise that only a proportion of B12 in the blood is 'active'.

Since the B vitamins and vitamin C are water soluble, unlike the other vitamins which are fat soluble, they are rarely found in excess in the body as the body simply excretes what it doesn't need. However, when the metabolism is at fault and/or fluid intake is low, it is possible to overload on vitamin B12 which could cause flushing, diarrhoea, nausea and vomiting.

Iodine

Due to the hormonal aspect of this disease, with the hypothalamus being affected by neurotoxins, many long COVID patients have been found to have thyroid problems.[15] This is compounded by the problem of iodine deficiency, which is a global issue.

In the early part of the 20th century, iodine deficiency was reduced by adding it to flour and salt. However, many people were found to be sensitive or allergic to iodine, with excess iodine resulting in thyroid inflammation. Therefore, in the 1980s it was removed from flour production and one rarely finds iodised salt now. In addition, over the last few years salt intake has reduced around the world.

A study in 2011 by the British Thyroid Association UK Iodine Survey Group showed that a high number of girls in the UK were iodine deficient.[16]

Iodine is an essential micronutrient. A deficiency is associated with goitre and hypothyroidism and pregnancy loss plus congenital anomalies and intellectual impairment in children born from iodine-deficient mothers.

Seaweed such as kelp is one of the best natural sources of iodine and can therefore be used to help some thyroid problems. However, it is not a good idea to overload the body with iodine for the reasons stated above, so don't have too much kelp. Advice from a nutritionist will be important.

Increased salt intake

The disturbed metabolism in long COVID can affect salt intake. Besides the iodine deficiency linked with reduced salt intake, sodium deficiency can produce an array of similar signs and symptoms to long COVID and is associated with a form of low blood pressure that occurs as one stands up after sitting or lying, called neurally-mediated hypotension (NMH). This drop in blood pressure corresponds with a drop in heart rate when tested on a tilt table.[17] However, although an increase in salt intake is advised for some patients, this may lead to severe, if not fatal, consequences if they suffer from high blood pressure generally. It is always best to check with the GP before increasing sodium in the diet.

Long COVID notoriously often overlaps with other medically unexplained syndromes due to the disturbed sympathetic nervous system, as detailed in Chapter 2. One of them is known as 'orthostatic intolerance' which refers to a group of clinical conditions in which symptoms worsen with upright posture and are reduced when lying down. The severe form of orthostatic intolerance is 'postural orthostatic tachycardia syndrome' (POTS) and this is discussed in more detail in Chapter 2 (page 57).

Essential fatty acids

Omega-3 and omega-6 fatty acids are hugely important in the regulation of inflammation and immune function. Long-chain omega-3 fatty acid EPA (eicosapentaenoic acid), which is mainly found in fish oils, helps reduce inflammation and is necessary for many biological processes in the body so it must be constantly replenished. Due to increased demands by long COVID patients and also the metabolic damage from viral infections, the patient usually doesn't have enough EPA, or enough of the anti-inflammatory omega-6 fatty acid GLA (gamma linolenic acid), which is found mostly in vegetable oils, especially evening primrose oil. Many people nowadays have a diet low in EPA but high in pro-inflammatory omega-6 AA (arachidonic acid) which in excess produces what is known as a low omega-3 index (the ratio between omega 3 and 6). This has been linked in ME/CFS patients to increased inflammation and the reduction of normal immune function,[18] aggravating symptoms of long COVID.

Central to the basis of the Perrin Technique™ is the fact that in long COVID the hypothalamus is overstimulated, leading to an overloaded autonomic nervous system. Nerves transmit their signal via chemicals known as neurotransmitters, as has been described. Too much of one of the main neurotransmitters, acetylcholine, breaks down into acetate and choline. Thus, when originally formulating my theory in 1989, I hypothesised that one day scientists would discover too much choline in the body.

An increase of choline was found in ME/CFS sufferers by Professor Basant Puri and colleagues at Hammersmith Hospital and Imperial College, London,[19] who also discovered a deficiency in fatty acids which are important for the healthy maintenance of cell membranes, especially in the brain.

Sometimes patients will have the opposite with a down-regulated hypothalamus, which I have seen in very severe patients. This could lead to a reduced autonomic control and a decrease in acetylcholine.

The same dysregulation of acetylcholine is happening with long COVID. Kopańska and colleagues firmly stated in their research review that COVID-19 causes a dysregulation of the cholinergic system which will alter the choline levels in the brain and cause dysregulation of the autonomic system, primarily the parasympathetic vagus nerve.[20]

It is of further significance that in a study by the Federation of American Societies of Experimental Biology into the effect of omega 3 fatty acids on the neuro-lymphatic/glymphatic system, there was better drainage from the brain to the lymphatics when the intake of omega 3 polyunsaturated fatty acids was increased.[21]

Guaifenesin

Guaifenesin is a pharmaceutical agent found in many cough medicines and is usually used as an expectorant, increasing the volume and reducing the viscosity of secretions in the passages of the lungs. It also has been shown to help relax muscles and has anticonvulsant properties. It is thought to do this by acting as an NMDA receptor antagonist.[22] In long COVID there is most likely in many patients an overactivity of the neurochemical NMDA in the thalamus of the brain due to neurotoxicity and so guaifenesin may help some of the symptoms. By reducing the action of NMDA it may help reduce the production of neuropeptide P which will help with pain. Plus, it may help with sinus congestion, which plagues many patients. Although there are no clinical trials to support its use in ME/CFS, I have known patients with the condition who have had relief from headaches and general aches and pains from taking this medication.

Adaptogens

Adaptogens are botanical medicines that have been used for centuries by eastern traditional medicine to help the body cope better with all forms of stress. Examples of adaptogens that have been shown to help long COVID patients include combinations of the adaptogens Rhodiola, Eleutherococcus, and Schisandra and may help reduce symptoms such as the duration of fatigue and chronic pain.[23]

Rhodiola rosea decreases cortisol levels in stress and reduces fatigue as well as increasing concentration.

Eleutherococcus senticosus (also known as Siberian ginseng) supports the adrenal glands and increases lymphocyte activity, helping the immune system. When I was heavily involved in sports medicine in the 1980s and 1990s, I used to treat many athletes who took Siberian ginseng to boost their performance, which was commonplace at that time. The World Anti-Doping Agency (WADA) classified ginseng as a permitted substance for athletes as it did not cause a positive doping test result. So, it may also help with energy in long COVID patients, but don't start trying to run the four-minute mile or the 100-metres in under 10 seconds.

Schisandra, (the magnolia vine), is a genus of twining shrub that in traditional Chinese medicine is used for many health issues including improvement of the body's immunity and aid sleep.

Other useful adaptogens that may help long COVID symptoms are:

Liquorice root has known antiviral properties.

Ashwagandha also has been shown to have good antioxidant properties aiding the immune and nervous systems and therefore helping the body cope better with stress.

Evidence supporting supplementation

There have been few randomised controlled trials of supplements specifically for long COVID but one of the first was conducted by Rathi and colleagues in 2021,[24] examining the effects of a combined enzyme and probiotic complex. They showed a significant reduction in both physical and mental fatigue which could be explained by the improvement of the microbiome's production of many neurochemicals needed by the brain.

Antihistamines

Dr Paul Glynne, a renowned specialist in long COVID, has revealed dysfunction of T-lymphocyte responses and inflammation, and a disturbed mast cell activation.[25] Mast cells are immune cells that release histamine and other chemicals. They are found in many places throughout the body, especially in the skin, lung airways and digestive tract, forming a first line of immunity, and throughout the body including the brain. They are most important for allergic responses and synthesise and secrete histamine.

Following certain stimuli they also produce and secrete many neurochemicals, such as the neuropeptide serotonin, and hormones, such as heparin needed for blood clotting, and many pro-inflammatory chemicals, such as prostaglandin, leukotrienes and a variety of cytokines. These three types of chemical are messengers that activate the immune response. They are molecules that are all formed from the breakdown of arachidonic acid (AA), a fatty acid component of cell membranes, and are important for the activation and production of inflammatory cells. Some classes of leukotrienes tighten the airway muscles and produce excess mucus during allergic reactions, causing the effects seen in asthma.

There are different types of antihistamine that have been produced over the years by the pharmaceutical industry. First-generation H1-histamine receptor antagonist antihistamines cross the blood–brain–barrier, and in usual doses can cause drowsiness and impair cognitive function. These antihistamines, such as chlorphenamine, are available over the counter in the UK as Piriton.

Second-generation H1-histamine receptor antagonist antihistamines do not pass the blood–brain–barrier and include loratadine, available in the UK over the counter as Clarytin. The more effective fexofenadine is often prescribed by GPs in the UK and is also selective for the H1 receptor but does not bind to off-targets that cause side effects.

Certain newer H2 histamine receptor antagonists such as famotidine (Pepcid) help promote gastric mucosal defences and are used in the treatment of acid-peptic disease, including duodenal and gastric ulcers, gastroesophageal reflux disease and common heartburn.

The overactivity of mast cells can lead to increased inflammation and persistent chronic inflammatory changes and the formation of fibrosis, autoimmune disease, micro-clots, gut dysbiosis, difficulty breathing and major neurological disturbance in both the central and peripheral nervous systems. This is why many doctors around the world are looking at mast cell activation syndrome as a major factor in the aetiology and pathogenesis of long COVID.

Dr Glynne has shared the benefits of his own observations, having treated over 300 long COVID patients. He has identified the major barriers to recovery from long COVID as including sleep disruption, stress and anxiety, overexertion, overworking and poor gut health and has focused on optimising sleep and pacing as important components of treatment.

Many of Dr Glynne's long COVID patients have responded extremely well to treatment with a combination of H1 and H2 receptor antagonists (antihistamines) which have the advantage that these drugs are safe and well tolerated.[25]

Sleep aids

As well as long COVID patients having sensitivities and/or allergies helped with antihistamines, many also have sleep disturbances as discussed in detail in Chapter 6. Therefore, I recommend first-generation antihistamines that cause drowsiness one hour before bed as this may 'kill two birds with one stone' – that is, help the sleep as well as the reduce the allergic reactions.

As many of the common foods we eat contain high levels of histamine I also recommend a low-histamine diet, avoiding the foods known to contain the highest levels of histamine such as tuna, mackerel, sardine and herring. Allowable meat and vegetables should be fresh. Grilling and frying may increase histamine in foods, so it is best to boil or bake foods when possible.

The plant valerian (*Valeriana officinalis*) has been used for thousands of years to aid sleep and grows wild in grasslands throughout North America, Asia and Europe. Researchers do not know exactly how it works but it is thought it could increase the gamma aminobutyric acid (GABA) in the brain; as we know, when the neuro-lymphatic system stops working, the GABA in the basal ganglia in the brain is affected.

The usual recommended dose is 300 to 600 mg of Valerian root 30 minutes to two hours before bedtime. Taking too high a dose of valerian root during the day can lead to daytime sleepiness. In 2006, Dr Stephen Bent and colleagues conducted a systematic review of 16 research studies showing evidence that extracts of the roots of valerian may improve sleep quality without producing major side effects.[26] Valerian root seems to work best after taking it regularly for two or more weeks but, as with all medication, even natural ones, you should always check with your doctor before taking anything I recommend to ensure it is right for you individually.

Antioxidants and immune support

One of the main types of lymphocyte that are part of the body's innate immune system are natural killer (NK) cells involved in the natural surveillance of any foreign invaders as well as any abnormal mutations of cells. They are important for detecting the development of cancer cells and are described by sleep scientist Matthew Walker as the 007s of the immune system as they seek out and destroy foreign invaders. NK cell activity has been shown to be supported by certain supplementation such as vitamin C,[27] which is a known antioxidant and also helps reduce mast cell overactivity. As mentioned earlier in the chapter, although many practitioners advise high doses of vitamin C, I recommend patients take 500 mg a day as a safe dose long term, to avoid too much calcium absorption in the body which can lead to the development of kidney stones.

Vitamin D, *Andrographis*, blackcurrant seed oil and zinc have also all been shown to help NK cell activity. *Andrographis paniculata*, also known as green chiretta is a plant native to India and Sri Lanka. It is widely used in southern and southeastern Asia and Africa as a treatment for bacterial infections and many other diseases.[28]

Other lymphocytes known as T-helper cells (also known as CD4+ cells) aid immune function by helping the action of NK cells, as well as helping the production of antibodies. These cells are suppressed in long COVID and T-helper cell activity has been reported by Yanuck and colleagues to respond well to supplementation such as quercetin, liquorice root, and astragalus.[29] However, a careful balance of these supplements is necessary as, if there is too much T-helper cell activity, it may exacerbate the effects of the inflammatory reflex where excess CD4+ cells could trigger a cytokine storm, leading to an autoimmune-like chronic neuro-inflammation via the gateway reflex.

Quercetin is a flavonoid, a plant pigment that contains the aromatic organic compound phenol and has existed in plants since prehistoric times. It is a potent antioxidant and is found mostly in onions, grapes, berries, cherries, broccoli and citrus fruits. Flavanols (a subset of flavonoids that include a ketone group in their structure) possess an ability to modulate the immune system by balancing the amount of T-lymphocyte activity.

Previous studies have demonstrated that flavonols reduce the risk of cardiovascular diseases, metabolic disorders and certain types of cancer. These effects are due to the physiological activity of flavonols in the reduction of oxidative stress, inhibiting LDL oxidation and platelet aggregation, and acting as vasodilators in blood vessels.[30]

I also recommend phytosterols, (also known as plant sterols), which are also found naturally in a variety of plants. Like cholesterol, they're a key structural component of cell membranes. Because phytosterols can block the absorption of cholesterol, they are often promoted as a way to improve heart health and decrease blood levels of the harmful LDL cholesterol.

Phytosterols, like flavanols, also help reduce the risk of disease by modulating the immune cells. They target specific T-helper lymphocytes, the Th1 and Th2 cells, helping normalise their functioning and resulting in improved T-lymphocyte and NK cell activity.[31]

Garlic is known for its antimicrobial properties. I usually advise patients with infections to take the highest dose possible of allicin. This is one of the active ingredients of garlic and has been shown to exhibit antibacterial activity against a wide range of gram-negative and gram-positive bacteria, which reduces the chance of secondary bacterial infection that could lead to pneumonia. Allicin has also been shown to promote antifungal activity, particularly against *Candida albicans*; antiparasitic activity, including against some major human intestinal protozoan parasites, and antiviral activity.[32]

If the allicin and phytosterols don't help I would advise the patient next to try echinacea – a good natural immune-system stimulant. Echinacea, also known as coneflower, is a native of central North America and used by native American tribes for sore throats, snake bites and sepsis. *Echinacea purpurea* is the most commonly used form. It seems to help the immune activity rather than target specific viruses. The recommended dose is usually in the region of 500 mg taken three times a day. However, echinacea shouldn't be used for more than a few weeks at a time; it is recommended only for short-term use.

One of nature's natural antibiotics, bee propolis, is also a useful tool when fighting infections.

Another very effective, but probably the most hideous-tasting natural remedy, is grapefruit-seed extract, which enhances the immune system and can be used to help with all manner of infections, whether parasitic, viral, bacterial or fungal. Grapefruit-seed extract has been shown to be effective at very low concentrations to reduce candida, and bacterial loads.[33]

WARNING: It is extremely important to realise that the list of adaptogens and supplements in this book are a general guide and not set in stone. Even herbal supplements and natural botanical products can have serious side effects, especially if combined with other prescribed medicines. For example, *Gingko biloba* and SSRI together may cause a potentially dangerous condition known as serotonin syndrome that is due to too much of the neurotransmitter serotonin. It is important to check with your doctor first before taking any products mentioned in this book to ensure that any drug interactions or chemical overloads are avoided in your individual case.

Conclusion

As the Roman poet and philosopher Lucretius (circa 94–55 BC) stated in *De Rerum Natura (On the Nature of Things)*[34]: '*Ut quod ali cibus est aliis fuat acre venenum*' – 'That which to some is food, to others is bitter poison'.

As shown in this chapter, as far as diet and nutritional aids go in long COVID, there are many approaches that may help, but on balance, I don't think there is one diet that works for everyone. I have included advice that |I have seen help in clinic with some long COVID patients or where the science backs up the claims. However, before you buy every supplement mentioned or give up your favourite foods, you should always consult with a qualified herbalist, nutritionist or doctor.

I usually advise long COVID patients to start small regarding any herbal remedy as many patients are highly sensitive to anything they put into their bodies. Consequently, starting with the lowest dose is always a good idea to help prevent any severe adverse reactions occurring. If even the lowest dose causes a problem, stop immediately and seek your practitioner's advice.

Chapter 10

24 hours in a life with long COVID: the dos and don'ts

'Oh don't go on like that!' cried the poor Queen, wringing her hands in despair. 'Consider what a great girl you are. Consider what a long way you've come today. Consider what o'clock it is. Consider anything, only don't cry!'

Lewis Carroll

Alice Through the Looking Glass and What Alice Found There

Case: Rebeka's story

Before I had COVID-19, I was an avid runner, worked a fast-paced job, and was busy with my three young kids. I just never stopped. But for the first time in my life, I didn't recover from this virus. Once the cough and fever went away, I got worse in other ways: I got weak and forgetful. I had to stop working and stay with my parents; I couldn't handle the sounds and activities at home. I ate meals fast, so I could lie back down after the effort of sitting up to chew my food. My sentences trailed off in confusion. I feared I might die and had mostly lost hope. My PCP (Primary Care Practitioner) had no idea how to help me.

After the first six weeks of the Perrin Technique™ treatment at the ME/CFS Clinic, I have been able to return home with my wife and kids. My arms now have the strength to do mom things like braid my daughter's hair. I am reading bedtime stories to the kids again. I've been able to be outside in the sunshine a little bit. I can talk without effort or losing my train of thought. Dr Tam is helping me plan my return to work now, and as the sole wage earner in my family, that's incredibly important.

I'm getting my life back! I know I still have a fair distance to go before I get back to a 'normal' life, but I am confident that, with support and guidance from Dr Tam, I will get there. She explained everything so well up front, and the process has gone just as she said it would. I know this treatment is a commitment and it's so worth the effort. Honestly, I'm still in awe that I'm actually recovering. Thank you to everyone who has made this clinic possible. My family and I are so grateful.

Rebeka McRad, Bloomington, MN, USA.
Patient of Osteopathic Physician and licensed Perrin Technique™ Practitioner Dr Ruby Tam DO, Minneapolis, USA

In this chapter I impart advice for long COVID patients on how best to get through each day and night, based on my decades of experience working with ME/CFS and FMS patients, backed up by the latest scientific findings from different experts in this field.

Morning routines

Waking up

Let us start with getting up in the morning. It should be morning, not after midday. This is very important, as getting into a reasonably normal sleep pattern is essential. One should aim at getting up every day, and even in severe cases one should try to wake up at the same time each day, preferably in the morning.

As explained in Chapter 6, the sleep–awake cycle is controlled by the hypothalamus, with the pineal gland in the brain which produces the hormone melatonin stimulated by the dark and suppressed by how much light passes through the eyes, which is why some people refer to the pineal gland as the 'third eye'. Dark and light stimulate the production of melatonin and serotonin, respectively. The melatonin/serotonin balance is crucial in maintaining a good diurnal rhythm and helping us stay awake during the day and sleep at night.

In the winter the darker days aggravate the rhythm, and some people suffer a drop in serotonin and become more depressed, leading to what is known as SAD (seasonal affective disorder). Also, many long COVID patients sleep much worse in the summer as they have too little melatonin and too much in the winter. To help the balance in winter, a SAD light which mimics daylight hours does often help. So, if you have this problem, a SAD light is important first thing in the morning at dawn for an hour, and another hour later on in the evening at twilight/dusk is also recommended.

Getting out of bed

If this is possible (and unfortunately, I have seen many patients who are unable to lift their heads off a pillow, never mind get out of bed), always alight from the bed in stages; never jump up as the control over blood pressure is often disturbed and experiencing dizziness when getting out of bed is common. So, before sitting up, make sure you are lying on your side and slowly swing your legs over the edge of the bed and gradually sit up at the side of your bed where you should remain for a minute or so before slowly standing up. If you suffer from POTS (postural orthostatic tachycardia syndrome – see page 57) you should stay seated for at least three minutes before trying to stand up.

Baths and showers

Water should never be too hot or too cold as the hypothalamus is the thermostat of the body and too extreme temperatures will stress an already overloaded part of the brain.

Try to avoid hot baths at any time. They are worse than showers as, besides overheating the body, the muscles will relax while the spine is in an unhealthy position unless you are able to float in the bath. It always amazes me as an osteopath how many people take a hot bath when they have lower back pain. Sitting in the bath places extra strain on the lower back and can aggravate any postural problem. With long COVID it is double trouble as the heat and the postural strain together exacerbate any inflammatory changes in the spine, which creates more toxicity within the central nervous system.

Comfortably cool baths that you can lie in are healthier for long COVID patients and sometimes relieve many of the symptoms, but if the water is too cold it will aggravate the condition by increasing tone in already tightened muscles. If you are going to try cool baths, make sure that when you are lying there you are not shivering and that you are comfortable. I recommend about 10 minutes at a time.

Showers are usually better for long COVID but if the patient feels dizzy or weak standing and does not have a bath then they should use a shower chair. If a patient constantly feels faint or actually faints in a hot shower and their heart rate frequently races, then again suspect possible POTS.

Having frequent short, cold showers of around 16–23°C may also be of benefit to some long COVID patients. As with cool baths, moderately cold showers have been shown to reduce pain by stimulating the production of endorphins which reduce pain without causing any harm.

Cool showers and baths have been shown to stimulate the locus coeruleus in the brain stem which forms a major axis, together with the hypothalamus, in the control mechanism of the neuro-lymphatic drainage system. In health this axis switches off during the night in deep restorative delta-wave sleep so, when this system is disrupted, it may have major consequences with the axis switching off at the wrong time leading to the patient feeling sick and exhausted as the toxins drain out of the brain during the day. To reverse this problem, we need to stimulate the locus coeruleus during the day. So, brief, comfortably cool hydrotherapy in the morning will greatly help some patients.

Exposure to cold typically causes activation of the sympathetic nervous system (SNS), which can cause problems with long COVID since the sympathetic nerves are usually overloaded. However, small amounts of stressful or harmful agents can sometimes be beneficial. This phenomenon is known as hormesis. Similar to the body's immune response needing to first be exposed to an infectious agent before it builds an immunity, as seen in vaccination, it is believed by some that exposure to cold can temporarily reverse autonomic dysfunction and therefore improve symptoms.

If your symptoms are improving with the manual therapy explained in this book but you wish to boost your energy, try the hydrotherapy once in the morning for just a few minutes, either lying in a cool bath or having bursts of a cold shower for a few seconds at a time over a couple of minutes. If it brings any relief, continue each morning so long as you always feel well afterwards. If it worsens your condition in any way, then immediately stop as it isn't for you. Remember that every long COVID patient is different, and unfortunately people respond differently to any stimulus.

On that note, there is a completely different form of hydrotherapy developed in Japan that has been shown to relieve mental fatigue. This is known as 'mild stream bathing' which involves a mild stream of warm water continuously passing from the sole to the calf, thigh, waist and back, providing a massage function. This form of therapy would stimulate lymphatic drainage, working against any backflow, so it may help long COVID as long as the water isn't too hot. It should only be attempted in the later stages of treatment as full body massage could easily overload the drainage of toxins and be too much for your body to cope with when embarking on the Perrin Technique™.

Make sure any soaps, shampoos and shower-gels are not too perfumed. Most perfumes and aftershaves should be avoided as they are made of petrochemicals and other ingredients such as phthalates and synthetic musks which can be neurotoxic. It is worth buying the least allergenic products recommended by your local pharmacist even if they are more expensive.

Clothes

Loose clothes that are easy to slip on and off are recommended as clothing that is too tight may restrict circulation of blood and lymph and lots of buttons etc can place strain on the hands that do get fatigued and sometimes become very painful. For women, tight bras are a definite no-no, especially tight underwired bras, which do place extra pressure on the breast lymphatics. Sports bras tend to be better, but the main issue is finding a properly fitted bra; bra-fitting services should be used and are available at good quality shops around the world.

Deodorants, antiperspirants and cosmetics

As with soaps, shampoos and shower-gels, most perfumed deodorants, antiperspirants and cosmetics should be avoided as much as possible, as they usually contain high levels of petrochemicals and other neurotoxins. There are safer products that are less toxic, but one has to shop around.

Mealtimes

Diets were discussed at length in Chapter 9, but the basic advice I give is not to eat anything in excess and generally, 'variety is the spice of life'. Eating a wide variety of foods generally places less strain on a particular part of the gastrointestinal system, which is often disturbed in long COVID patients, with many having irritable bowel syndrome (IBS) and gut dysbiosis.

Dietary intake of sugar should be low as it stimulates the production of yeast. Patients with long COVID should eat less casein (found in milk-based products), less gluten, as well as less yeast, as these are all composed of large molecules and therefore require the lymphatics to drain the excess away from the gut.

Small meals eaten regularly are best and I often advise patients to drink 2 litres of water a day, either on its own or in healthy drinks such as herbal caffeine-free teas. Patients should reduce the intake of caffeinated coffee and tea as caffeine can over-stimulate the nervous system.

As explained in Chapter 9, alcohol should be avoided at all costs. This is because, beside it obviously placing extra strain on the liver, when it reaches the brain it will affect the neurochemicals NMDA and GABA, which are both prolific in the regions of the brain first affected by any neuro-lymphatic disturbance, i.e. the thalamus and the basal ganglia respectively. Most of my patients do not find this advice difficult to follow as they feel worse even after a little sip and almost drunk following the smallest amount of alcohol.

Daytime routines

During the day and especially at night, the long COVID patient has to learn how to relax and possibly meditate. A new word has been coined that embodies both relaxing and remaining chilled and calm: 'chillax'. There are plenty of different strategies to do this, including mindfulness. If you are having difficulty getting to sleep, relaxation and/or meditation is essential, or just do a relaxing activity such as listening to soft music (not heavy metal) or a talking book (not of the horror or thriller genre).

Bedtime routines

Difficulty falling asleep and staying asleep, known as insomnia, and hypersomnia, when the patient sleeps too much, and other sleep disturbances, are very common symptoms of long COVID – see Chapter 6 for the science behind this. Leading sleep experts, including Dr Jason Ellis, Professor of

Sleep Science and Director of the Northumbria Sleep Research Laboratory in the UK, advocates cognitive behavioural therapy for insomnia, often called CBT-I.

CBT-I is an approved method for treating insomnia aimed at changing sleep habits and includes regular, often weekly, visits to a clinician and completing a sleep diary to work out the best way of tackling the specific disorder.

Sleep clinics around the world offer many ways of analysing the sleep problem and for those patients with severe sleep disorders a polysomnography test is essential. Also known as a sleep study test, polysomnography records your brain waves, the oxygen level in your blood, heart rate and breathing, as well as eye and leg movements.

As mentioned plenty of times in this book, exertive exercise should always be avoided, even when on the path to recovery from long COVID. However, if you are fit enough to take part in some aerobic exercise such as walking, cycling or swimming, always avoid exercising in the last three hours before going to bed.

On the other hand, exercises to help you to fall asleep should be attempted, such as counting backwards from a thousand … in sevens – i.e. 1000, 993, 986, 979 etc. It isn't easy and that is the main point. By taking your mind off everything else your brain will be calmer and you will gently fall asleep. At the same time, it can also help if you think 'I am not going to sleep … I am not going to sleep' and repeat this over and over again in your mind while counting down from 1000 in 7s.

It is best to have a set bedtime and stick to it as closely as possible. A very good idea recommended by sleep expert Matthew Walker is to set an alarm to remind you to go to bed. In fact, there are many wellness apps available that automatically send you this reminder.

Use blackout curtains and switch off all lights in the room. It's best to take all electronic gadgets away from the bed. Avoid tea, coffee and any other drinks with caffeine before bedtime. In fact, caffeine's stimulating effects can take about eight hours to wear off so it's best to avoid any caffeinated drinks in the late afternoon as well as the night time.

Some patients find a warm bath before bed helps as, when they get out of the water, their body naturally cools and this helps sleep. Make sure your room is never on the hot side. Cool is much better for good sleep so experiment and then keep the temperature of your room at the level that gives you the best night's sleep.

A good mattress is so important as we spend almost a third of our lives in bed … or we should do! (My patients will call me a hypocrite for recommending this, but as I tell them every day … 'Do as I say … not as I do'!). I always recommend a mattress with as many pocket springs as possible to give good support to the body. Go into the bed shop/showroom and try out the mattresses before you buy the bed. Lie on many different beds and choose the one that feels most comfortable. There is an osteopathic adage – 'comfort governs function' – so if it doesn't feel right it's going to harm your sleep.

Sometimes having a small meal an hour before bed helps. As most people have experienced, after a heavy meal during the day, one often feels very drowsy. This is because hormones released after eating can also stimulate the sleep centres. These hormones are controlled by the hypothalamus which is, as we have seen, the main part of the brain disturbed in long COVID. Eating food can calm the hypothalamus and help induce sleep.

However, make sure the pre-sleep meal isn't too large as it can cause indigestion which can definitely affect sleep, especially if gastric reflux is a problem. Try also to avoid too much fluid intake before bed as it will increase the need to urinate in the middle of night.

Alcohol should always be avoided as mentioned earlier, but some patients who can't sleep may think that a 'wee dram' before bed will help sleep. Alcohol can reduce the quality of sleep, affecting neurotransmission, especially during REM sleep.

As discussed in Chapter 9, valerian root has been used since ancient times as a herbal remedy to aid sleep. It has helped many patients and there are several valerian root products on the market today; however the amount of valerian root in capsules available varies widely.

If you do wake up at night, do not just lie there in bed listening to the snoring of your partner or wondering what time it is and worrying about what you have in store the next day. Get up and go to the toilet if need be and then, in a warmly lit room, have a caffeine-free drink and a little snack, such as a piece of toast (gluten-free if possible) have a little read of the newspaper (as long as there is some good news) or a book and after about half an hour go back to bed and use some of the CBTi methods mentioned at the beginning of this section.

The benefits of fresh air

So, with these tips and understanding sleep and the difficulties long COVID presents, you should be able to sleep for longer at the right time and have better quality sleep, allowing you to wake up more refreshed.

As soon as you are up and about, following the steps at the beginning of this chapter you should, if possible, go outside in the daylight and get the sun's rays to shine on you, stimulating serotonin and breathing fresh air, especially if you live near a forest or wooded region, which will be richer in oxygen, giving you a further boost of energy. The air we breathe outside contains only around 20% oxygen (this is 'normal' – that is, what our lungs have evolved to work with), but this is reduced inside the home, so if you/the long COVID-sufferer is bedridden then ventilate your/their room as much as possible.

In the summer, or throughout the year in warmer climates, this could be coupled with 'earthing', which is walking barefoot on grass or sand, allowing your body to earth electromagnetic energy it receives from our planet (see Chapter 8).

Conclusion

My techniques, like all forms of medicine, are not the Holy Grail, able to help all, and my heart goes out to any patient who is not benefiting from the advice and treatment in this book. However, Perrin Technique™ practitioners across the world are improving the health of the majority of their patients, which is all I could ever expect.

The Perrin Technique™ is not a miracle cure but it addresses a necessary pathway of the lymphatic drainage of the central nervous system that has been ignored by most of the medical world for centuries and I believe is an essential part in the jigsaw puzzle of health, especially in diseases where the main factor is a dysfunction of the neuro-lymphatic drainage, such as long COVID.

I do hope that, after reading this book, you have found the information helpful in understanding this illness that is affecting millions around the world. Most people when they understand my theory and methods of diagnosis and treatment say: 'Well, that makes sense'. As English biologist Thomas Huxley famously said: 'Science is nothing but trained and organised common sense.' However, most importantly, if you have long COVID yourself I do very much hope that this book will help you on the road to recovery.

To this end, the Appendix which follows has been written for patients and practitioners to be able to quickly answer common queries and to help people with long COVID manage their illness and aid recovery.

Appendix

Frequently asked questions

Case: Hollie's story

When I first met my Perrin Technique™ practitioner, Michael Parr, I had been suffering with COVID-induced fatigue for three years and had recently given up my job. I had started to experience fatigue after my first COVID vaccine in 2021. I was an otherwise healthy and active 26-year-old, but I reacted relatively badly to the vaccines, with heavy flu-like symptoms and a chesty cough. Throughout the summer, I was fighting through a strange fog of tiredness, dizziness and feeling lightheaded. I thought I might be a bit unfit so leant into activities like tennis and swimming. Over the course of the next couple of years my symptoms worsened; I caught COVID in March 2022 and found it difficult to recover. I was tired all the time and never felt refreshed, no matter how much I rested. I experienced headaches and dizziness which worsened to migraines; sometimes I felt unable to move due to the discomfort. I stopped sleeping and developed depression. I really didn't know what was wrong with me; I concluded it was probably long COVID-related, but I thought I was healthy and didn't understand why I felt so unwell.

I had contacted Michael a couple of weeks prior to quitting my job regarding mild scoliosis and chronic pain in my neck. I mentioned to him in passing that I thought I had chronic fatigue, at which point he told me that he also treated patients with ME/CFS using the Perrin Technique™. I had never heard of this technique before, but I felt such a sense of relief that someone could finally confirm that I wasn't well, I wasn't making this up in my head, and that they could do something to help.

I was given a rough timeline for recovery which allowed me to see an end goal. Without this hope, I am not sure how I would have coped. I carried out self-massage once daily from the beginning of my treatment; Michael taught me one element per week which made it feel manageable. This gradual approach to adding in treatment and exercise has definitely allowed me to stay consistent and now it all feels like second nature to me.

At first, I felt like my fatigue was worsening; I had stopped all activity and was being cared for by my parents as I was unable to cook for myself, carry out any household chores, drive etc. My body had been pushed to the absolute limit and had finally been given the chance to crash. When I had particularly severe periods of fatigue, Michael was always able to explain the cause: drainage in my lymphatics, excessive heat in the summer, anxiety and stress or my menstrual cycle, which worsened my symptoms every month. This attention to detail and expertise gave me a real feeling of reassurance and empowerment. I started taking supplements, getting blood tests and improving my diet to target my deficiencies, which also gave me agency to do something positive towards my recovery.

I am really happy to say I have seen a gradual improvement in my symptoms over the last year. I can get quite anxious and often doubt whether I will recover, so holding on to even tiny improvements is very important for me. I see a therapist who really helps me to try and live happily within my limits. Gradually, I've felt a little less exhausted and more able to leave the house. I can do my rehab exercises to improve alignment on a regular basis and I've started to feel bored, which is a good thing as it sees me itching to do more! Sometimes I still overdo things, and my activity is limited, but as long as I stay within my limits and am consistent with the Perrin Technique™ routine, my rest periods are shorter, and I rarely feel completely wiped out.

This treatment has helped improve all aspects of my physical and mental health; I've learnt new techniques and habits that should lead to a healthier life. I am a calmer person now with a positive outlook and I am starting to plan for my future again.

Hollie Drinkwater, Cambridge, UK
Patient of osteopath and licensed Perrin Technique™
practitioner Michael Parr, Elementary Health, UK

How much exercise and activity can I do?

I am still shocked to hear of some long COVID patients around the world being encouraged by their doctor to do more and more exercise in a bid to improve their health.

As discussed in Chapter 2, post-*exertion* malaise (PEM) is one of the most common symptoms in long COVID … not post-*exercise* malaise. Any activity that does not over-exert you will be okay and activity is encouraged, if possible, as long as it does not exhaust you. PEM may not be immediate; the malaise may kick in up to three days following exertion, so beware of this problem. Also, it is important also to realise that PEM relates not only to physical exertion but also to mental.

It is best to avoid all exertive exercise and sport until you are virtually symptom free and then you can revitalise your deconditioned body by gradually increasing your activity.

Rehabilitation and reconditioning patients' weakened bodies has to be done safely, for example using the back sculling swimming stroke described in Chapter 7 (Fig. 43). As the symptoms continue to improve, both the patient and the practitioner will be greatly encouraged. By steadily improving the mobility of the spine, and by relaxing all the irritated surrounding tissues, the function of the sympathetic nervous system should finally be restored to full working order. The patient once again enjoys health, vigour and a good quality of life and hopefully can go back to a more active lifestyle exercising in gyms and playing sports.

However, … never forget my golden rule for any activity – what I call the 'half rule', i.e. only do 50% of what you feel capable of.

The 'half rule' is so difficult to adhere to because, once on the mend, it is as though your prison door has been unlocked for the first time in maybe years and yet you are only allowed to walk around the courtyard and then go back into your cell. However, if you were to run out of the prison gates too quickly, the guns and dogs of long COVID would be there ready to stop you, the fleeing prisoner, in your tracks. Much better to walk calmly out through the gates at a very gentle pace and then stop and return for a while and then go a bit further the next time, continually returning to the safety of the cell for a while. This allows you to slowly but surely leave the long COVID prison without alerting the sympathetic nervous system's 'prison guards' and finally escape their clutches.

Patients who are eager to resume some form of aerobic exercise and can't swim, or live too far from a swimming pool or suitable beach, or remain sensitive to chlorine, should begin by gentle walks up and down the street and gradually increase the distance. Walking should be on the flat at the beginning of rehabilitation and, if possible, while wearing a pedometer, which is a device that counts each step a person takes by detecting movement of the arms or hips; this is a very useful tool to monitor the gentle progress that you should be aiming for.

A pedometer can simply be downloaded as an app for your phone or you can buy a simple device in most sports supply shops. Gradually increase the activity, keeping to walking and not jogging: shifting all one's weight onto first one side and then the other places too much strain on the spine whereas walking avoids this jarring effect.

Cycling should only be done on the flat. As with walking, avoid hills to begin with as this may over-exert your back and leg muscles. A basic exercise bike with a little resistance is also a good form of rehabilitation.

REMEMBER: graded activity does not help long COVID patients recover but helps re-condition the recovered patient!

What hobbies can I do safely?

Hobbies and pastimes are very important for patients' sense of purpose and sanity, especially if housebound. They can also be a crucial part of rehabilitation, reintroducing physical and mental activity to a life that has just been about existing from day to day. If the hobby involves arts and crafts, the patient may be suffering neurotoxicity from the paint, paint thinners and solvents they use. These and many other hobbies involving toxins should be kept to a minimum for obvious reasons. Patients should wear a mask if there is any danger of exposure to poisonous fumes.

Playing a musical instrument is a favourite among some patients as they increase their capabilities. This is highly recommended, but again try to space out the sessions whatever instrument you enjoy playing, and when playing the piano, to begin with, use a supportive chair rather than a standard piano stool as sitting with no back support will place extra strain on your spine.

If recovering patients take to gardening, they have to be careful not to expose themselves to organophosphates, such as pesticides and herbicides. Also, patients should invest in tools with long handles that reduce the need to stretch and bend. Be careful when carrying out repetitive actions to prevent overstraining weakened muscles.

Is technology safe to use?

People always think watching TV is a very passive activity and cannot overload the nervous system. They couldn't be more wrong. TV images create a hive of neuronal activity in the brain as one has to digest what is going on in each scene of a play, film or even a gameshow or the news. Screens also send out 'blue light', which has been shown to stimulate alpha-waves (see page 161). During the morning, blue light is beneficial as it boosts mood, reaction times and concentration, but in the evening, and especially just before bed, it reduces good restorative sleep, so the advice to all patients is: do not watch TV for at least an hour before bed. A survey by a leading phone manufacturer found that almost nine out of 10 18–34-year-olds have trouble sleeping because they use their smartphones at bedtime.[1] Technology firms have acknowledged the problem, with some major mobile tech providers introducing special settings that reduce blue light. Special yellow or orange tinted glasses can also be used to filter out the harmful blue light.

Blue-light-filter glasses or blue-light-filter apps should definitely be used if using a computer for long periods. Many of my younger patients spend much of their day playing on computer games or looking at their phones. These screens should be set up with filters that shield the blue light as the day draws to a close. As with TV, all screens should be avoided for an hour before bed even when using the filter.

I recommend listening to relaxing music, reading a book that is in the light-reading genre (i.e. not a thriller or horror story) or, if reading is difficult, listening to a talking book last thing at night as a good alternative.

Any screen-time should be restricted during the day as spending too long in one position can lead to postural strain on the spine and repetitive strain injuries when using game consoles or texting. Muscles are much more susceptible to damage from constant repetitive trauma, especially in FMS. Hands-free options and non-metal cases on phones should be used to reduce radio frequency exposure.

When can I return to work/education?

If you have been off sick from work for a protracted amount of time, as you improve and are well enough to start work, you should never consider just returning to work full-time as soon as you feel better. You need to gradually increase hours in a phased return-to-work programme, such as that shown in Table A. The phased return schedule depends on many factors and differs from patient to patient. This is an example of a recommended schedule I have used in clinic.

The phased return schedule depends on many factors and differs from patient to patient. The rule of thumb is that you should listen to your body and symptoms. In other words, if you are struggling mid-way through the phased return programme and find four hours a day too much, you can go back a week or two in the schedule.

A similar situation occurs when a young patient is out of full-time or part-time education due to long COVID. Pressure to place the young person back into school is often compounded by social services becoming involved. Parents continue to be suspected of making their child worse than they actually are. Conditions like 'Munchausen's syndrome by proxy' and 'fictitious illness syndrome' have been mentioned by the authorities, at times accusing patients' parents of making their children feel ill without any real physical cause of the disease.

Once the young person begins to improve, they can return to school, maybe just at break-time to begin with, so that there is some social interaction with

Table A. Example of a phased return to work programme

Week	Monday	Tuesday	Wednesday	Thursday	Friday
1	1 hour		1 hour		1 hour
2	2 hours		2 hours		2 hours
3	3 hours		3 hours		3 hours
4	4 hours		4 hours		4 hours
5	4 hours		4 hours		4 hours
6	4 hours		4 hours		6 hours
7	6 hours		4 hours		6 hours
8	6 hours		6 hours		6 hours
9	6 hours		6 hours		8 hours
10	8 hours		6 hours		8 hours
11	8 hours		8 hours		8 hours
12	8 hours		8 hours	2 hours	8 hours
13	8 hours		8 hours	4 hours	8 hours
14	8 hours		8 hours	6 hours	8 hours
15	8 hours		8 hours	8 hours	8 hours
16	8 hours	2 hours	8 hours	8 hours	8 hours
17	8 hours	4 hours	8 hours	8 hours	8 hours
18	8 hours	6 hours	8 hours	8 hours	8 hours
19	8 hours	8 hours	8 hours	8 hours	8 hours

their peer group. Little by little, add an extra class into the phased return schedule, and as long as the young person feels that they are not getting too tired, they should continue to build-up their attendance.

University courses often present a problem as one cannot usually attend full-time degrees in a part-time capacity unless one joins a part-time course. This should sometimes be considered if the illness is too severe to continue. Another alternative is for severe patients to defer their university place for a time and hopefully they will be able to return to their studies once recovered. This has been the case with many of my student patients and most go on to receive a much better degree than if they had tried to struggle through. I am so proud of many of my patients who have deferred their university course and end up with excellent final exam results, going on to flourishing careers.

Are there any dos and don'ts on commuting?

Travelling to and from work and school should always be factored into any phased return. Any travelling that places the patient under too much strain should be avoided. Going by train for long distances is usually better than driving as sitting for long periods can easily harm the spine. On the train the patient can get up and walk around a little as well as have a rest without the extra stress of traffic jams.

If I am improving, can I go on holiday?

When you are well enough to take a vacation, it shouldn't first be a long-haul flight to a country that is very hot. Patients need to shelter from too much sun. Symptoms of long COVID are exacerbated by jet lag, excessive temperatures and sunburn.

Often it's not the holiday that harms the patient, and a beach with fresh air and some sun and shelter, with the occasional dip into the sea, is often the best place to be. The problem lies in getting there and airports with their queues, and the long distances to the gate can be very damaging to the patient.

So, when flying I always advise patients who haven't yet recovered to order wheelchair support at airports. However much the patient may dislike the public display of their illness, they never regret following this advice since most airport staff look after wheelchair passengers and their families really well and take all the stress out of the airport experience.

If you have to go on a long-haul flight that may induce jet lag, ask your doctor or pharmacist about melatonin to take after the long flight, especially one that is travelling eastwards, such as from the USA to Europe. Melatonin helps to regulate the body's circadian rhythm and helps some patients' sleep problems. It is prescribed off-label for jet lag in many countries, but it is best to ask your doctor's advice before taking it.

When on holiday in a hot climate, make sure you keep in the shade as much as possible and use the highest-rated sunblock. Sunburn will aggravate the pain in long COVID, so you need to avoid direct sun when possible. Try to avoid overheating and going to winter resorts that are too cold, as both will strain your hypothalamus, which is the body's thermostat, as discussed earlier. The best option is to go on vacation where the weather isn't too extreme.

It isn't just the temperature that can affect a long COVID patient. It may be that the amount of light during the day can have a major effect on the symptoms due to the melatonin/serotonin balance when patients suffer from seasonal affective disorder (SAD) worsening the condition in the darker winter months (see Chapter 10). This can be remedied by using a SAD light and obviously not going to a holiday destination that is in mid-winter if you do have these problems.

It is not only the time of the year affecting seasonal changes that may be a problem for some patients. It is an interesting fact that some of my patients with long COVID seem to worsen at certain times of the month and it is not just women due to their menses cycle. The time of the month that patients worsen sometimes follows the lunar cycle, with the occasional patient reporting worse symptoms during a full moon. Just throwing an idea out to the reader, and as discussed earlier, there may be a scientific reason for this happening in long COVID as well as other neuro-lymphatic disorders as discussed next.

The moon has a major effect on the tides due to its gravitational pull. If this celestial body can exert its influence on the oceans, it is surely going to have some effect on the comparatively minute amount of fluid draining out of the brain. Therefore, I believe that in some cases, a full moon may increase the backflow pulling toxins into the brain and worsening some symptoms. So, if you are one of those patients, don't think you are losing your mind and you are definitely not a werewolf, but more sensitive to the gravitational pull of the moon, which is greater midway through a lunar month.

Is it safe to get pregnant with long COVID?

Women with long COVID should assess their own state of health before embarking on a pregnancy. The effects of pregnancy on long COVID are unknown at present but women with fatigue and breathlessness can expect a deterioration during pregnancy, especially in the third trimester.[2]

However, many long COVID cases are similar to ME/CFS so I will give some guidance based on ME/CFS in pregnancy. There are two viewpoints concerning pregnancy and ME/CFS. Some experts believe that pregnancy is a time when a better balance is achieved within the woman's body, and it can help reduce the symptoms of ME/CFS. Some healthy women blossom when pregnant; if the long COVID patient is lucky enough to be that type, her symptoms will probably reduce during pregnancy.

However, this is unpredictable, if the mother-to-be is one of those individuals who generally have a difficult pregnancy, her long COVID symptoms may worsen for most of the nine months as her hormone levels fluctuate, producing more nausea and fatigue.

A case report in a leading journal also warned that deteriorating symptoms during pregnancy and in postnatal long COVID mothers should be fully evaluated before being ascribed to long COVID. The paper stresses that additional support from family, friends and healthcare professionals is paramount.[2]

No large studies have yet been done on long COVID pregnancies. However, a study published in 2004 showed that symptoms improve in about one third of pregnant ME/CFS patients, usually after the first trimester, and are unchanged in about one third, and worsen in about one third, with worsening symptoms in their second and later pregnancies.[3]

Long COVID presents a problem for the actual delivery of the baby as the natural pain in childbirth will be exacerbated and aggravate the widespread pain due to the illness. Gas and air or hypnosis should be considered before opting for any other forms of analgesia for the birth itself.

From a positional point of view, the best position for patients giving birth is the left lateral position, which is still commonly used and reduces strain on the spine compared with any other position.

If local or general anaesthetics are used in the labour, then one should check that they are safe and are non-adrenaline (-epinephrine) based.

If there is a choice between having a spinal block/epidural or electing to have a Caesarean section, I would opt for the latter as injecting an anaesthetic directly into the spine is definitely not recommended for patients with long COVID due to its neurotoxic properties. Also, with discovery of the SLYM (page 150), the membrane of the brain and spinal cord dividing the subarachnoid space from healthy cerebrospinal fluid and the toxic drainage from the brain, there is a big risk with any needles entering the spine damaging this very fragile film.

It is important to make sure that any supplements as well as medication taken for long COVID should be confirmed by your doctor as safe to take during pregnancy.

It's not just the pregnancy; it's the baby afterwards that obviously places more strain on the mother, and this is more of a problem. In moderate to severe cases I would usually advise a patient to wait until they have recovered before getting pregnant.

Breastfeeding carries the risk of toxins being transferred from mother to baby, so the best advice regarding this factor is for the mother to have as much detox treatment as possible before she plans on getting pregnant.

If I require surgery, what precautions are needed?

You may have other problems that require an operation. If surgery is not essential, I would advise a delay as long as possible until you have improved with my treatment. However, occasionally surgery is crucial and needs to be done as soon as possible. In these cases, the advice I give to patients about general anaesthetics is that the anaesthetist should be aware of the illness and to follow the advice given to ME/CFS patients by of one of the leading experts in this field, American physician Dr Charles Lapp.

Some patients have low magnesium and potassium levels so Dr Lapp recommends pre-operative tests for serum magnesium and potassium should be done as low levels can affect the heart under anaesthesia.

Many long COVID patients, especially the very severe, housebound patients, have a problem with their hypothalamic–pituitary–adrenal axis affecting their adrenal glands. Therefore, Dr Lapp also advises that cortisol levels should be tested before any operation on ME/CFS patients, as low levels could place the patient at risk, so supplements may be required before surgery can commence. Also, if a local anaesthetic is used in any procedure, it should be non-adrenalin based. This is the same with long COVID.

All supplements should be discussed with the anaesthetist to check that they will be safe to take and that they will not interfere with the surgery or the anaesthetic. If possible, it is usually sensible to avoid most supplements for two weeks before surgery, especially garlic, ginseng and *Gingko biloba*, which increase bleeding.

Most of my long COVID patients have managed to recover quite quickly post-surgery, as long as they have taken things very easy and convalesced after their ordeal. The days of convalescent homes are long gone but, when patients return home from hospital, they should be very careful to pace their activity to avoid a relapse of their symptoms.

How important are environmental factors?

All of us are exposed to a number of pollutants in our everyday lives. Long COVID sufferers need to minimise as far as possible their exposure to these toxins.

Sometimes it is not patients themselves who are directly exposed to a pollutant or environmental toxin. It can often be a family member who may be an engineer, hairdresser or car-paint sprayer as examples of particularly toxin-related jobs. Many patients have had a possible neuro-lymphatic drainage problem since birth and have been harmed by living in a household where one or both parents have jobs that bring them into increased contact with toxins. The parents come home and may hug their baby and wash their clothes in the same machine as their child's clothes. This cross-contamination over the years can lead to the gradual build-up of neurotoxins in the brain and spinal cord, with the child eventually having sufficient exposure to trigger the onset of long COVID. Sometimes the onset of illness will be many years later when the patient is an adult. Medicines for babies and children are given in minimal dosages since the young are much more susceptible to the effects of toxins, illustrating the fact that in the young toxic exposure does not have to be great to inflict harm.

When visiting the dentist, avoid having mercury amalgam dental fillings. When going to have your hair done at the hair salon, the use of chemicals in your hair should be limited, especially since some have been shown to harm the actual hairdresser. Remember that the scalp is very close to the brain, and it is not advisable to massage poisons into the skin in this area. Take care to make sure that your neck is in a comfortable position, too, when your hair is being washed in a back basin.

Patients who are hairdressers themselves, or in other occupations that use large amounts of toxic materials, should take extra measures to avoid further exposure, such as wearing gloves and masks and having plenty of ventilation. This is advice that is all too familiar from life in the midst of the COVID-19 outbreak, but any patient working with toxins should continue to take these measures in the post-pandemic era.

If you live in the countryside, take a trip away from home during crop spraying days. If your work entails exposure to harmful toxins, you may need to consider a career change.

Many of my patients relax by lighting scented candles at home. Unfortunately, aromatic candles are nearly all highly toxic, with the wax usually having a high petrochemical content and the wicks usually containing heavy metals. In January 2024, Dr Tamás Pándics, a public health specialist at Semmelweis University in Hungary, went public in the world press stating: 'We expose ourselves to the effect of hundreds of substances which, with the additional unnecessary burden of substances such as scented candles, home fragrances and wall-plug-ins, can lead to serious problems'.[4] If you enjoy candles to relax, please try and use beeswax ones with natural, non-metallic wicks.

If you move into a new home and you have new carpets, curtains and other soft furnishings, make sure you have plenty of ventilation. When decorating, use low-odour paint and again it is best to stay out of the house when the paint is being applied, especially the gloss. Make sure any home gas appliances are not emitting harmful carbon monoxide; ensure that you have detectors fitted in your home. Also, if you live in a damp, older property have an environmental check for mould.

When using mobile phones, make sure you use a hands-free option as much as possible as holding it close to the head has been shown to damage the blood–brain–barrier, making the brain more vulnerable to toxins.

Can the Perrin Technique™ help with other conditions?

This is a tricky question to answer. The simple answer is yes. Over the years, I have had the wonderful pleasure of working alongside some amazing doctors. One is leading neurologist Dr Margareta Griesz-Brisson in Harley

Street, London. She always says: 'Ray, we are treating the physiology, not the pathology.' In other words, the treatment is designed to aid the restoration of a healthy neuro-lymphatic system, which physiologically will encourage the central nervous system to work better. So, many problems affecting the nervous system should be helped by the Perrin Technique™.

There are other diseases linked to problems affecting the lymphatic drainage of the brain. Scans in 2012 by a group of neuroscientists in Rochester University in New York State revealed visible proof of the drainage of beta-amyloid proteins out of the brains of mice via the perivascular spaces into the lymphatic system. This showed how these large molecules could stagnate in diseases such as Alzheimer's, which has been linked to the accumulation of beta-amyloid plaques and Tao protein molecules, which destroy connections between the brain's neurones, affecting thinking, memory and behaviour.[5]

In his new book *Dispatches from the Land of Alzheimer's*[6] Dr Danial Gibbs, a retired neurologist who has Alzheimer's, reveals changes in his lifestyle that have helped him live with this progressive disease and that have definite neuro-lymphatic links. He talks about high cholesterol links with Alzheimer's and how reducing cholesterol helps. The lymphatics should control excess cholesterol by draining it away from the GI tract in the chyle, but if there is a disturbed sympathetic control of the central lymphatics then the excess cholesterol will flow back into the tissues, including the spinal cord and the brain, causing too much cholesterol in the brain and thereby creating inflammatory changes in the microglia.

Dr Gibbs also found that drugs known as acetylcholinesterase inhibitors may help. These medicines stimulate an increase of acetylcholine which is a major neurotransmitter for the parasympathetic and sympathetic nervous systems. He also found that exercise and activity help in most cases, especially if aerobic exercise routines are started before the onset of the main symptoms of the Alzheimer's. This is where the diseases differ. Long COVID is not helped by exercise and often there are higher levels of acetylcholine in the brain so, although I believe that the diseases are both due to a reversal of the lymphatic system control, with Alzheimer's there is a secondary vascular challenge leading to the symptoms of dementia. Aerobic exercise and increased blood flow will help these patients. However, in most cases of long COVID the primary problem is the backflow of the glymphatics that may be worsened by too much acetylcholine and definitely by doing too much exercise, so one has to be cautious in not treating all neuro-lymphatic diseases the same. However, improved glymphatic drainage will most definitely help and the sooner the better, before the brain is too damaged.

The Rochester University group have also shown that the neuro-lymphatic system is dependent on two factors:[7]

1. Pressure differences between intracranial blood pressure and the adjacent glymphatic system's pressure allowing cerebrospinal fluid to be pushed through tissues.
2. High blood pressure and intercranial pressure aggravated by tension together with the reduction of delta-wave sleep affects the glymphatic drainage.

I have treated a few patients with Alzheimer's disease and one elderly man in the early stages of the disorder received once-a-month treatment for four years with no deterioration in his symptoms throughout the four years. In fact, he sometimes came in for his monthly session saying he had had the best month yet, with increased energy and concentration and memory as good as ever. Sadly, he subsequently had a fall and injured his head which led to a speedy deterioration in his condition.

Another condition that I have helped many patients with over the years is Lyme disease; with this infection, the reverse flow of lymphatic drainage leads to a build-up of the bacterium *Borrelia burgdorferi* in the central nervous system. Research has also shown that problems with lymphatic drainage of the brain may also lead to some forms of clinical depression and rarer conditions such as Creutzfeldt-Jakob disease (CJD) caused by a build-up of proteins known as prions. A genetic defect can lead to another rare condition causing a mass spread of prion proteins, especially in the thalamus, that causes destruction of the sensory gate allowing a permanent opening into the brain of all sensory inputs that eventually stops the patient from sleeping completely. This is known as fatal familial insomnia (FFI). If the neuro-lymphatic system worked better, severe fatal conditions like CJD and FFI might be helped and who knows possibly eradicated in the future.

Lymphoedema and lipoedema

One of the roles of the lymphatic system is to drain away excess fluid that may build up in the tissues. If this function is compromised, it can lead to swelling in the body known as lymphoedema. (In the USA, it is written as 'lymphedema' (without the 'o').)

Most cases of lymphoedema are secondary following damage or pressure to the lymphatic vessels or lymph nodes and are generally unilateral, i.e. affecting one side of the body. Although lymphoedema can be the consequence of treatment for any cancer that involves removal of lymph nodes or damage of lymph vessels from radiation treatments, this disorder is most often recognised associated with breast cancer treatment specifically. For instance, after a mastectomy and removal of the axillary lymph nodes in the armpit, the arm on the side of the surgery may swell due to disruption of the lymphatics in that body region. Treatment, including manual lymphatic drainage and compression therapy, will be required for the rest of the patient's life in order to properly manage the swelling (oedema) and maintain the health of the affected arm.

Other causes of secondary lymphoedema are blocked or slowed drainage due to tumours that press on lymph vessels or parasites that burrow into the lymphatic vessels. Filarial worms and their larvae are parasitic thread-like round nematodes transmitted to humans through a mosquito bite, causing filariasis (philariasis).[8] This parasitic disorder, most common in Africa and southern Asia, is also known as elephantiasis because of the disfigurement and large size of the legs, often due to poor access to proper treatment.

Primary (hereditary) lymphoedema is considered a rare condition and affects both sides of the body, but asymmetrically. Swelling can be present at birth, but most commonly tends to start at puberty (lymphoedema praecox or Meige's syndrome) or at other times of hormonal change, such as pregnancy or menopause (lymphoedema tarda). This, along with the greater prevalence in females, strongly suggests a hormonal influence.[9]

Peripheral lymphoedema is confirmed by the Kaposi-Stemmers Sign (better known as just 'Stemmer sign').[10] A positive sign is demonstrated by the inability to pinch and lift the skin at the base of the dorsum of the second toe or finger. The difficulty in lifting tissue suggests oedema and skin thickening that is characteristic of lymphoedema.

Lipoedema (also spelled in the USA without the 'o') is another lymphatic disorder that presents as an abnormal build-up of fat, predominantly in the lower body but can occur in the arms. Lipoedema affects women almost exclusively. Other symptoms include pain and easy bruising in the affected body areas, distinctive tissue changes such as fatty nodules and fibrosis, and oedema (swelling). Lipoedema and lymphoedema can co-occur, a condition which is sometimes referred to as lipo-lymphoedema.

The hypothalamus is under more pressure in menstruating women due to cyclical hormonal changes and also during periods of major hormonal flux such as puberty, pregnancy and menopause. This factor is one of the main reasons why women suffer more from long COVID, ME/CFS and fibromyalgia syndrome and may be a major aetiological factor in primary lymphoedema and lipoedema.

I believe that lymphoedema and lipoedema are due to the resultant central sympathetic nerve dysfunction leading to a backflow of lymph, eventually creating oedematous changes in some patients who may have inherent weaknesses in their lymphatic system. In many of these patients, there is also a reversal of flow of chyle, the creamy white lymphatic fluid present in the intestinal lymphatics. Chyle is full of glycoprotein molecules known as chylomicrons (see Chapter 9) containing harmful long-chain triglycerides. The backflow will lead to deposits of fat in many different parts of the body, contributing to the creation of the swollen and painful fatty lumps that cause misery for so many women around the world.

There is even a recognised condition known as generalised lymphoedema associated with neurologic signs (GLANS) syndrome.[11] This syndrome is almost certainly due to the lymphatics of the central nervous system being compromised and therefore should be helped by the Perrin Technique™.

The Perrin Technique™ can most definitely help in improving the central lymphatic drainage in patients with lymphoedema and lipoedema. It is highly recommended that this is performed in conjunction with specialised treatment from a trained manual lymphatic therapist or a practitioner of complete decongestive therapy (CDT), a treatment developed in the early 1980s by Professors Michael and Etelka (Ethel) Foëldi of the Foëldiclinic in Hinterzarten, Germany.

Just a few weeks before completing the first draft of this book I had the honour to spend a long weekend in Cambridge, Massachusetts where I met up with an amazing group of practitioners and patients who are part of a worldwide network focusing on lymphoedema and lipoedema.

Lipedema Simplified is the brainchild of its founder and CEO Dr Catherine Seo, who has started treatment with one of my trained practitioners in the USA and is already starting to benefit. Catherine was introduced to my work by a patient, Kelly Bell, who was an engineer and a retired US Coast Guard. Below is the email he sent to Catherine in August 2023 when the group first heard about my work; it highlights the importance of treating the lymphatics using the Perrin Technique™ for lymphoedema and lipoedema.

Case: Kelly's story

In May 2005 … I received a treatment called 'ENTERYX' for acid reflux/hiatal hernia (later determined a misdiagnosis). ENTERYX is a plastic/polymer bulking agent that is made by mixing ethylene vinyl alcohol copolymer, DMSO and tantalum powder (which is why you can see it in the attached images). The product is no longer used to treat hiatal hernias. As you can imagine, I slowly developed a number of issues. In 2007, a CT was performed and the polymer was noted to be in my liver, spleen, lungs (especially right) and possibly heart. An endoscopic ultrasound a few weeks later confirmed the polymer was in the lymph nodes of my liver. In 2008, I had surgery to remove some of the polymer that was accidentally pushing my vagus nerve. During the surgery, it was discovered that the middle lobe of my right lung had turned fibrotic and it was removed along with hilar lymph nodes, subcarinal mediastinal lymph nodes, and lower mediastinal lymph nodes. It was also confirmed there was polymer in the lymphatics on my heart. The surgeons also discovered the tantalum did not mix with all the polymer because it was noted in the lymphatics and tissue and was opaque and not black. The polymer could not be safely removed from any of the tissues without causing damage so it remains.
The surgery only resolved a few issues, and slowly I started having pulmonary, kidney, cardiac, GI, liver and neurologic issues.

In 2010, I had an upper and lower lymphoscintigraphy and it was noted after a full day of scanning that contrast had only made it to my cisterna chyli. (See Fig 46). I was asked to return the next morning and the contrast had not progressed at all after 24 hours of scanning. So, my next question was, 'How do the nutrients from the thoracic duct get to my organs?' Still no answer to that question. A researcher presented during the 'Yet to be charted: Lymphatics in Health and Disease' conference from NIH last year that some chyle leaks from the mesenteric lymphatics, into the endothelial cells and over to the liver, basically requiring

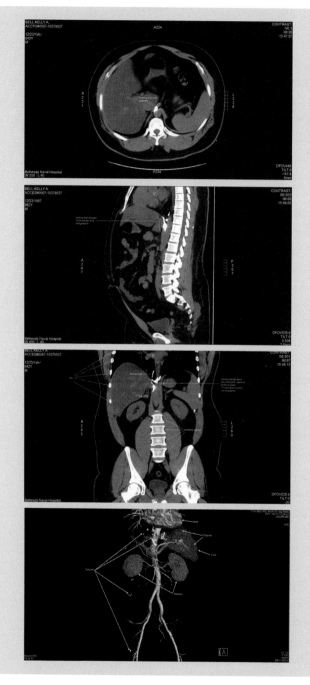

Fig. 46 Axial, sagittal, coronal and 3D rendition of CT scans showing polymer in central lymphatics.

my portal vein and liver to handle the full fat load creating inflammation in them. My health was on a downward trajectory until 2017 when I discovered that the main source of fuel to function, heal and grow for the lymphatics were fats and went on a ketogenic diet. It worked really well for about two years, and then slowly quit working. I surmise after the information I learned from the NIH conference that it was because my liver and portal vein began to struggle handling the fat load.

Last year, after presenting at a lymphedema conference, the right side of the back of my head swelled and I began having issues with memory and putting words together and tears began running from mainly my right eye. I went to the ER and a CT was performed and it showed lymph nodes were swollen on the right side and back of my head and neck but nothing else was noted. MRI three weeks later diagnosed microvascular ischaemic disease and early-onset Alzheimer's. I have had swelling under the right side of my chin and sometimes to a small extent at the back of my head since 2005. The back of my neck is always swollen with fluid to varying degrees. My abdomen is always swollen. My BP is on average 121/78 mm Hg. Resting pulse is 55 bpm on average. I currently weigh 273 pounds [124 kg]. I have to use a CPAP and monitor my breathing with a pulse/ox at night. Always fighting energy issues and crazy headaches now.

Since we aren't dealing with biologics in me and the plastic isn't going anywhere, we do focus on moving fluid throughout my entire trunk and head. We (my wife and I) are getting things to move in the right direction again, slowly. I know how lymphatics work and they are always making new channels. The issue I keep running into is when I get something going, it apparently stops and I have to build another one. I am constantly running labs to make certain the things I am doing aren't putting any stress on my organs and working on lowering inflammatory markers.

I am still amazed where Dr Perrin was in the early 90s and to know a lot of what he hypothesised has been proven. Any ideas or just a chance to pick his brain would be fantastic.

Thanks again!

Kelly A Bell, LT
Oak Island, North Carolina, USA
US Coast Guard (ret)

Since the above email sent in August 2023, Kelly's health has steadily been improving after he received regular sessions of the Perrin Technique™ with a trained practitioner in North Carolina where he lives with his therapist wife, Jen, who is now herself a trained licensed Perrin Technique™ practitioner.

Californian occupational therapist and expert lymphoedema therapist Dr Leslyn Keith is president of the Board of Directors for the Lipedema Project also set up by Catherine Seo, a non-profit organisation dedicated to raising awareness, providing education, and supporting research to identify treatment and a cure for lipoedema and teaches lymphatic therapy. She has authored a few books and her latest excellent gem, *The Lymphatic Code*, delves into the latest facts of the anatomy and physiology of the lymphatics, explaining the role of the lymphatics in health and disease and explains lymphoedema and lipoedema in superb detail plus looking at all diets used to help lymphatics an extols the ketogenic diet to improve the overall health of the lymphatic system.[12]

As the lymphatic drainage of the brain is being further investigated by neuroscientists around the world, more conditions will probably be connected to the dysfunction of this important process. This will probably indicate the validity in using the techniques shown in this book to treat many other diseases, neurological and otherwise that, at the time of writing, have no successful treatment and continue to baffle the medical world.

Once I have recovered, can the illness recur?

As patients recover, if they overdo things, suffer from infections or have to cope with too much stress, their symptoms may return or worsen. Some patients do suffer recurrences after they have significantly improved, but few experience relapses once they have been discharged, unless they push themselves too far day after day. Long COVID patients, once recovered, need to reassess their lifestyle and take steps to reduce the continual stress that may have been part of what led to the illness in the first place. One should be able to exert oneself when better, but knowing when to stop is important.

Patients who have been discharged should continue the dorsal rotation exercises (pages 185) three times a day for life. Self-massage to the chest and neck should be done once a week in the shower. An annual check-up is advisable.

Should a relapse occur, it may take a long time to reverse, but remember that, if the treatment worked the first time, it should work again and perhaps more quickly the second time. Psychologists and counsellors are invaluable in these cases. The important rule in treatment, and even more so after relapse, is to remain as positive as possible. Negative thoughts create further neurotoxicity.

To secure a permanent remission and to remain in good health, one has to focus on the task ahead by means of sensible pacing (the '50% rule'), thus achieving a slow but sure return to good health.

Following a graded exercise programme, but only when better, is a good idea, not to treat the long COVID itself, but to help recondition the body and to remain fit and well in the future.

Can long COVID be prevented?

I am one of the few practitioners who maintain that ME/CFS and FMS can be prevented and I feel the same with long COVID. The physical signs are very real and usually are seen long before the symptoms begin. This is why in the very early stages of the disorder only a physical and postural-based examination can detect the development of these disorders before the sympathetic nervous system breaks down.

If long COVID is found in more than one family member, there is probably a genetic predisposition that leads to a restricted flow of toxins from the brain and spine. I have discovered when examining children, siblings or even parents of the patient that they present some or all of the five physical signs of long COVID (see Fig. 1, Chapter 2).

When treating pre-ME, as I call it, the signs significantly reduce, usually with only a few weeks or months of treatment. For this reason, I believe that ME/CFS is preventable if treated and managed properly in the early stages. The same can be said for long COVID.

The very severe cases of patients in bed all day and night in silent, darkened rooms should never happen, as early diagnosis should then be followed up quickly with advice on pacing and the appropriate treatment, as was shown in a pilot study my research colleagues and I ran in 2022.[13]

The severe cases may be as a result of the wrong treatment or bad advice being given in the early stages of the illness, with patients being instructed and sometimes coerced to increase their activity, and sometimes medicated with drugs that have severe effects on the central nervous system.

If all practitioners around the world were taught to examine patients for the early physical signs of neuro-lymphatic disorders such as long COVID, which are evidence-based, and to carefully review the patient's history and symptoms for indications and signs of neurotoxicity, there would be far fewer severe cases. If patients were given advice to pace at the outset, together with prompt treatment to restore a healthy neuro-lymphatic system, it could help prevent long COVID developing in the first place, and one day make this and other similar terribly cruel illnesses a thing of the past.

References

Chapter 1   Long COVID: What's really going on?

1. Perrin, R., Riste, L., Hann, M., Walther, A., Mukherjee, A. and Heald, A. (2020) 'Into the looking glass: post-viral syndrome post COVID-19', *Med. Hypotheses*, 144:110055. DOI: 10.1016/j.mehy.2020.110055
2. Callard, F., Perego, E. (2021) 'How and why patients made Long Covid', *Soc. Sci. Med.*, 268:113426. DOI: 10.1016/j.socscimed.2020.113426
3. Nath, A. (2020) 'Long-haul COVID', *Neurology*, 95(13): pp. 559-560. DOI: 10.1212/WNL.0000000000010640
4. NICE (2020, updated 2024) *COVID-19 rapid guideline: managing the long-term effects of COVID-19*. NICE guideline [NG188]. Available at: https://www.nice.org.uk/guidance/ng188 (Accessed: 2 May 2024).
5. Centers for Disease Control and Prevention (CDC) (2023) *International Classification of Diseases, Tenth Revision, Clinical Modification (ICD-10-CM)*. Available at: https://www.cdc.gov/nchs/icd/icd-10-cm.htm (Accessed: 2 May 2024).
6. International Classification of Diseases (2024) 'RA02 Post COVID-19 condition', *ICD-11-CM*. 11th edn. Available at: https://icd.who.int/browse/2024-01/mms/en#2024855916 (Accessed: 13 May 2024).
7. The World Health Organization (WHO) (2024) *Post COVID-19 condition (Long COVID)*. Available at: https://www.who.int/europe/news-room/fact-sheets/item/post-COVID-19-condition (Accessed: 2 May 2024).
8. US Department of Health and Human Services (2024) *Long COVID or Post-COVID Conditions*. Available at: https://www.cdc.gov/coronavirus/2019-ncov/long-term-effects/index.html (Accessed: 13 May 2024).
9. Medinger, G., Altman, D. (2022) *The Long Covid Handbook*, London: Penguin Random House, p. 7.
10. Office for National Statistics (ONS) (2023) *Prevalence of ongoing symptoms following coronavirus (COVID-19) infection in the UK*, 30 March. Available at: https://www.ons.gov.uk/peoplepopulationandcommunity/healthandsocialcare/conditionsanddiseases/bulletins/
11. Hughes, S.E., et al. (2022) 'Development and validation of the symptom burden questionnaire for long covid (SBQ-LC): Rasch analysis', *BMJ*, 377: e070230.

DOI: 10.1136/bmj-2022-070230

12. Jason, L.A., Islam, M.F. (2022) 'A classification system for Post-Acute Sequelae of SARS CoV-2 Infection', *Central Asian Journal of Medical Hypotheses and Ethics*, 3(1), pp. 38–51.

13. Carruthers, B.M., van de Sande, M.I., De Meirleir, K.L. *et al.* (2011) 'Myalgic encephalomyelitis: international consensus criteria', *J. Intern. Med.*, 270(4): pp. 327–338. DOI: 10.1111/j.1365-2796.2011.02428.x

14. Fineberg, H.V., Brown, L., Worku, T., Goldowitz, I (Eds) et al. *The 2024 NASEM Long COVID Definition*. National Academies of Sciences, Engineering, and Medicine; Health and Medicine Division; 11 June 2024. https://nap.nationalacademies.org/resource/27768/Long_COVID_Definition_Highlights.pdf (Accessed 8 July 2024)

15. Porges, S.W. (2009) 'The polyvagal theory: New insights into adaptive reactions of the autonomic nervous system', *Cleve. Clin. J. Med.*, 76(Suppl 2), pp. S86–S90. DOI: 10.3949/ccjm.76.s2.17

16. Tracey, K.J. (2007) 'Physiology and immunology of the cholinergic anti-inflammatory pathway', *J. Clin. Invest.*, 117(2), pp. 289–96. DOI:10.1172/JCV130555

17. Tanaka, Y. *et al.* (2017) 'The gateway reflex, a novel neuro-immune interaction for the regulation of regional vessels', *Front. Immunol.*, 8, p. 1321. DOI: 10.3389/fimmu.2017.01321

18. Proal, A.D. and Van Elzakker, M. (2021) 'Long COVID or post-acute sequelae of COVID-19 (PASC): an overview of biological factors that may contribute to persistent symptoms', *Front. Microbiol.*, 23, p.12:698169. DOI: 10.3389/fmicb.2021.698169

Chapter 2   Diagnosing long COVID

1. Grisanti, S.G., *et al.* (2022) 'Neurological long-COVID in the outpatient clinic: Two subtypes, two courses', *J. Neurol. Sci.*, 439, p. 120315. DOI: 10.1016/j.jns.2022.120315

2. Niazkar, H.R., Zibaee B., Nasimi, A., Bahri, N. (2020) 'The neurological manifestations of COVID-19: a review article', *Neurol. Sci.*, 41(7), pp. 1667–1671. DOI: 10.1007/s10072-020-04486-3

3. Gasser, H.S. (1955) 'Properties of dorsal root unmedullated fibres on the two

sides of the ganglion', *Journal of General Physiology*, 38(5), pp. 709–728. DOI: 10.1085/jgp.38.5.709

4. Kinmonth, J.B. (1982) *The Lymphatics*. 2nd edn. London: Edward Arnold, p. 80.

5. Kinmonth, J.B. (1960) 'Some aspects of cardiovascular surgery', *Journal of the Royal College of Surgeons of Edinburgh*, 5, pp. 287–297.

6. Kinmonth J.B., Sharpey-Schafer, E.P. (1959) 'Manometry of human thoracic duct', *J. Physiol. (Lond.)*, 145, p. 3.

7. Vodder, E. (1936) *Le drainage lymphatique, une nouvelle méthode thérapeutique*. Paris, France: Santé Pour Tous.

8. Browse, N.L. (1968) 'Response of lymphatics of canine hind limb to sympathetic nerve stimulation', *Journal of Physiology*, 197(1), pp. 25–36. DOI: 10.1113/jphysiol.1968.sp008542

9. Still, A.T. (1899) *Philosophy of Osteopathy*. Kirksville, MO: published by the author.

10. Still, A.T. (1902) *The Philosophy and Mechanical Principles of Osteopathy*. Kansas City, MO: Hudson-Kimberly, p. 47.

11. Sutherland, W.G. (1939) *The Cranial Bowl*. Mankato, Minnesota: Free Press Company.

12. Sutherland, W.G. (1990) *Teachings in the Science of Osteopathy*. Edited by A.W. Wales. Fort Worth, TX: Sutherland Cranial Teaching Foundation.

13. Perrin, R.N. (2007) 'Lymphatic drainage of the neuraxis in chronic fatigue syndrome: a hypothetical model for the cranial rhythmic impulse', *Journal of the American Osteopathic Association*, 107(06), pp. 218–224.

14. Dreha-Kulaczewski, S. *et al.* (2015) 'Inspiration is the major regulator of human CSF flow', *Journal of Neuroscience*, 35(6), pp. 2485–2491. DOI: 10.1523/JNEUROSCI.3246-14.2015

15. Jänig, W., Levine, J.D., Michaelis, M. (1996) 'Interactions of sympathetic and primary afferent neurons following nerve injury and tissue trauma', *Progress in Brain Research*, 113, pp. 161–184. DOI: 10.1016/s0079-6123(08)61087-0

16. Marsden, C.D., Merton, P.A., Morton, H.B. (1973) 'Is the human stretch reflex cortical rather than spinal?', *Lancet*, 1(7806), pp.759–761. DOI: 10.1016/s0140-6736(73)92141-7

17. Perrin, R.N., Richards, J.D., Pentreath, V., Percy, D.F. (2011) 'Muscle fatigue

in ME/CFS and its response to a manual therapeutic approach: a pilot study', *International Journal of Osteopathic Medicine*, 14(3), pp. 96–105. DOI: 10.1016/j.ijosm.2010.12.002

18. He, J., Hollingsworth, K., Newton, J., Blamiria, A. (2013) 'Cerebral vascular control is associate with skeletal muscle pH in chronic fatigue syndrome patients both at rest and during dynamic stimulation', *Neuroimage Clin.*, 2, pp. 168–173. DOI: 10.1016/j.nicl.2012.12.006

19. Natelson, B.H., Vu, D., Coplan, J.D., Mao, X., et al. (2017) 'Elevations of ventricular lactate levels occur in both chronic fatigue syndrome and fibromyalgia', *Fatigue: Biomedicine, Health & Behavior*, 5(1), pp. 15–20. DOI: 10.1080/21641846.2017.1280114

20. Appleman, B. *et al.* (2024) 'Muscle abnormalities worsen after post-exertional malaise in long COVID', *Nature Communications.*, 15(1), p. 17. DOI: 10.1038/s41467-023-44432-3

21. Cervia-Hasler, C. *et al.* (2024) 'Persistent complement dysregulation with signs of thromboinflammation in active Long Covid', *Science*, 383(6680), p. eadg7942. DOI: 10.1126/science.adg7942

22. Farooqui, A.A., Farooqui, T., Sun, G.Y. *et al.* (2023) 'COVID-19 blood lipid changes, and thrombosis', *Biomedicines*, 11(4), p. 1181. DOI: 10.3390/biomedicines11041181

23. Van Ness, J.M., Snell, C.R., Stevens, S.R. (2007) 'Diminished cardiopulmonary capacity during post-exertional malaise', *J. Chronic Fatigue Syndr.*, 14, pp. 77–85. DOI: 10.1300/J092v14n02_07

24. Jason, L. *et al.* (2015) 'The problems in defining post exertional malaise', *J. Prev. Interv. Community*, 43(1), pp. 20–31. DOI: 10.1080/10852352.2014.973239

25. Carruthers, B.M., van de Sande, M.I., De Meirleir, K.L. *et al.* (2011) 'Myalgic encephalomyelitis: international consensus criteria', *J. Intern. Med.*, 270(4), pp. 327–338. DOI: 10.1111/j.1365-2796.2011.02428.x

26. Chu, L., Valencia, I.J., Garvert, D.W. and Montoya, J.G. (2018) 'Deconstructing post-exertional malaise in myalgic encephalomyelitis/ chronic fatigue syndrome: A patient-centered, cross-sectional survey', *PLoS One*, 13(6), p. e0197811. DOI: 10.1371/journal.pone.0197811

27. Torjesen, I. (2020) 'NICE advises against using graded exercise therapy for patients recovering from COVID-19', *BMJ*, 370, p. m2912.

DOI: 10.1136/bmj.m2912

28. Stone, W. (2024) 'A discovery in the muscles of long COVID patients may explain exercise troubles', *Shots Health News from NPR*, 9 January. Available at: https://www.npr.org/sections/health-shots/2024/01/09/1223077307/long-covid-exercise-post-exertional-malaise-mitochondria (Accessed: 3 May 2024).

29. Perrin, R., Riste, L., Hann, M., Walther, A., Mukherjee, A., Heald, A. (2020) 'Into the looking glass: post-viral syndrome post COVID-19', *Med. Hypotheses*, 144:110055. DOI: 10.1016/j.mehy.2020.110055

30. Lu, R., Zhao X., Li, J. et al. (2020) 'Genomic characterisation and epidemiology of 2019 novel coronavirus: implications for virus origins and receptor binding', *Lancet*, 395(10224), pp. 565–574. DOI: 10.1016/S0140-6736(20)30251-8

31. 31. Moldofsky, H., Patcai J. (2011) 'Chronic widespread musculoskeletal pain, fatigue, depression and disordered sleep in chronic post-SARS syndrome; a case-controlled study', *BMC Neurol.*, 11, p. 37. DOI: 10.1186/1471-2377-11-37.

32. Hives, L., Bradley, A., Richards, J. *et al.* (2017) 'Can physical assessment techniques aid diagnosis in people with chronic fatigue syndrome/myalgic encephalomyelitis? A diagnostic accuracy study', *BMJ Open*, 7(11), p. e017521. DOI: 10.1136/bmjopen-2017-017521

33. Kida, S., Pantazis, A., Weller, R.O. (1993) 'CSF drains directly from the subarachnoid space into nasal lymphatics in the rat. Anatomy, histology and immunological significance', *Neuropathol. Appl. Neurobiol.*, 19(6), pp. 480–488. DOI: 10.1111/j.1365-2990.1993.tb00476.x

34. Montoya, J.G., Holmes, T.H., Anderson, J.N., *et al.* (2017) 'Cytokine signature associated with disease severity in chronic fatigue syndrome patients', *Proc. Natl. Acad. Sci.*, 114(34), pp. E7150–E7158. DOI: 10.1073/pnas.1710519114

35. Carruthers, B.M., van de Sande, M.I., De Meirleir, K.L. *et al.* (2011) 'Myalgic encephalomyelitis: international consensus criteria', *J. Intern. Med* 270(4), pp. 327–338. DOI: 10.1111/j.1365-2796.2011.02428.x

36. Davis, H.E., McCorkell, L., Vogel, J.M., Topol, E.J. (2023) 'Long COVID: major findings, mechanisms and recommendations', *Nat. Rev. Microbiol* 21(3), pp. 133–146. DOI: 10.1038/s41579-022-00846-2

37. Ray, C., Weir, W.R.C., Phillips, L., Cullen, S. (1992) 'Development

of a measure of symptoms in chronic fatigue syndrome: the profile
of fatigue related symptoms (PFRS)', *Psychol. Health* 7, pp. 27–43.
DOI:10.1080/08870449208404293

38. Heald, A.H., Perrin, R., Walther, A. *et al.* (2022) 'Reducing fatigue-related
    symptoms in long COVID-19: a preliminary report of a lymphatic drainage
    intervention', *Cardiovasc. Endocrinol. Metab* 11(2), p. e0261.
    DOI: 10.1097/XCE.0000000000000261

39. Wostyn, P. (2021) 'COVID-19 and chronic fatigue syndrome: Is the worst yet to
    come?', *Medical Hypotheses* 146, 110469.
    DOI: 10.1016/j.mehy.2020.110469

40. Long Covid Moonshot (2024) *Join the movement*. Available at:
    https://longcovidmoonshot.com (Accessed: 3 May 2024),

41. Johnson, C. (2024) 'The Long COVID Moonshot Blasts Off (Without ME/CFS/
    FM, Lyme, POTS, etc.)', *HealthRising*, 18 April 2024. Available at: https://
    www.healthrising.org/blog/2024/04/18/the-long-covid-moonshot-blasts-off-
    without-me-cfs-fm-lyme-pots-etc/ (Accessed: 3 May 2024).

42. Agarwal, A.K. *et al.* (2007) 'Postural orthostatic tachycardia syndrome',
    Postgrad. Med. J 83(981), pp. 478–480.
    DOI: 10.1136/pgmj.2006.055046

43. Jacob, G. and Biaggioni, I. (1999) 'Idiopathic orthostatic intolerance and
    postural tachycardia syndromes', *Am. J. Med. Sci.*, 317(2), pp. 88–101.
    DOI: 10.1097/00000441-199902000-00003

44. Rowe, P.C. *et al.* (1999) 'Orthostatic intolerance and chronic fatigue syndrome
    associated with Ehlers-Danlos syndrome'. *J. Pediatr.*,135(4), pp. 494–499.
    DOI: 10.1016/S0022-3476(99)70173-3

45. Kokorelis, C., Malone, L., Byrne, K., Morrow, A., Rowe, P.C. (2023) 'Onset
    of postural orthostatic tachycardia syndrome (POTS) following COVID-19
    infection: a pediatric case report', *Clin. Pediatr. (Phila.)*, 62(2), pp. 92-95. DOI:
    10.1177/00099228221113609

46. Hoad, A., *et al.* (2008) 'Postural orthostatic tachycardia', *Quarterly Journal of
    Medicine* 101(12), pp. 961–965. DOI: 10.1093/qjmed/hcn123

47. Freeman, R., *et al.* (2011) 'Consensus statement on the definition of orthostatic
    hypotension, neurally mediated syncope and the postural tachycardia
    syndrome', *Auton. Neurosci* 161(1–2), pp. 46–48.
    DOI: 10.1016/j.autneu.2011.02.004

48. Low, P.A (ed.) (2000) *Orthostatic Intolerance*. National Dysautonomia Research Foundation Patient Conference; Minneapolis, Minnesota, USA; 2000.

49. Medows, M.S. *et al*. (2019) 'The benefits of oral rehydration on orthostatic intolerance in children with postural tachycardia syndrome'. *J. Pediatr* 214, pp. 96–102. DOI: 10.1016/j.jpeds.2019.07.041

50. Pollack, B. *et al*. (2023) 'Female reproductive health impacts of Long COVID and associated illnesses including ME/CFS, POTS, and connective tissue disorders: a literature review', *Front. Rehabil. Sci.*, 4, p. 1122673. DOI: 10.3389/fresc.2023.1122673

51. Beighton, P.H., Solomon, L., Soskolne, C.L. (1973) 'Articular mobility in an African population', *Ann. Rheum. Dis.*, 32(5), pp. 413–418. DOI: 10.1136/ard.32.5.413

52. Heffez, D.S. (2011) 'Is Chiari-I malformation associated with fibromyalgia? Revisited', *Neurosurgery*, 69(2), pp. E507. DOI: 10.1227/NEU.0b013e3182214cea

53. Higgins, J.N.P., Pickard, J.D., Lever, A.M.L. (2017) 'Chronic fatigue syndrome and idiopathic intracranial hypertension: different manifestations of the same disorder of intracranial pressure?' *Medical Hypotheses* 105, pp. 6–9. DOI: 10.1016/j.mehy.2017.06.014

54. Higgins, N., Pickard, J., Lever, A. (2013) 'Lumbar puncture, chronic fatigue syndrome and idiopathic intracranial hypertension: a cross-sectional study', *JRSM Short Rep.*, 4(12), p. 2042533313507920. DOI: 10.1177/2042533313507920

55. Hulens, M. *et al*. (2018) 'The link between idiopathic intracranial hypertension, fibromyalgia, and chronic fatigue syndrome: exploration of a shared pathophysiology'. *J. Pain Res.* 11, pp. 3129–3140. DOI: 10.2147/JPR.S186878

56. Thakur, S. *et al*. (2023) 'Covid 19 Associated idiopathic intracranial hypertension and acute vision loss'. *Indian J. Otolaryngol Head Neck Surg* 75(2), pp. 1031–1034. DOI: 10.1007/s12070-022-03303-x

57. Silva, M.T.T., Lima, M.A., Torezani, G., *et al*. (2020) 'Isolated intracranial hypertension associated with COVID-19'. *Cephalalgia* 40(13), pp. 1452– 458. DOI: 10.1177/0333102420965963

58. Reitsma, S., *et al*. (2007) 'The endothelial glycocalyx: composition, functions, and visualization'. *Pflugers Arch* 454(3), pp. 345–359.

DOI: 10.1007/s00424-007-0212-8

59. Sahin, M., Akkus, A. (2021) 'Fibroblast function in COVID-19', *Pathol. Res. Pract* 219, p. 153353. DOI: 10.1016/j.prp.2021.153353

Chapter 3   The role of toxins in long COVID

1. 'Toxin' (2001) *The New Oxford Dictionary of English*. Oxford: Oxford University Press.

2. Glynne, P, Tahmasebi, N, Gant, V, Gupta, R. (2022) 'Long COVID following mild SARS-CoV-2 infection: characteristic T cell alterations and response to antihistamines'. *J Investig Med* 70(1): 61–67.
    DOI: 10.1136/jim-2021-002051 PMCID: PMC8494538

3. Lazarus, M, *et al.* (2007) 'EP3 prostaglandin receptors in the median preoptic nucleus are critical for fever responses.' *Nat Neurosci* 10(9): 1131–1133.

4. Brierley, SM, Hibberd, TJ, Spencer, NJ. (2018) 'Spinal afferent innervation of the colon and rectum'. *Front Cell Neurosci* 12: 467.

5. Breit, S, *et al.* (2018) 'Vagus nerve as modulator of the brain–gut axis in psychiatric and inflammatory disorders'. *Front Psychiatry* 9: 44.
    DOI: 10.3389/fpsyt.2018.000440

6. Holzer, P. (2016) 'Neuropeptides, microbiota and behavior'. *Int Rev Neurobiol* 131: 67–89.

7. Tilson, H.A., Mitchell, C.L. (1992) *Neurotoxicology*. New York: Raven Press.

8. Sabljic, A. (1991) 'Chemical topology and ecotoxicology'. *Sci. Total Environ* 109–110, pp.197–220. DOI: 10.1016/0048-9697(91)90178-H

9. Cribb, J. (2017) *Surviving the 21st Century: Humanity's Ten Great Challenges and How We Can Overcome Them*. Cham, Switzerland: Springer International.

10. Rogers, S. (1990) *Tired or Toxic*. Syracuse, New York: Prestige Publishing.

11. Hanin, I. (1996) 'The Gulf War, stress and a leaky blood-brain barrier', *Nature Medicine* 2(12), pp. 1307–1308. DOI: 10.1038/nm1296-1307

12. Witte, S.T., Will, L.A., Olsen, C.R., Kinker, J.A., Miller-Graber, P. (1993) 'Chronic selenosis in horses fed locally produced alfalfa hay'. *Journal of the American Veterinary Medical Association* 202(3), pp. 406–409.

13. Schwarz, B., Salak, N., Hofstotter, H., Pajik, W., Knotzer, H., Mayr, A., Hasibeder, W. (1990) 'Intestinal ischemic reperfusion syndrome: pathophysiology, clinical significance, therapy'. *Wien Klin. Wochenschr* 111(14), pp. 539–548.

14. White, J.F. (2003) 'Intestinal pathophysiology in autism'. *Exp. Biol. Med.* 228(6), pp. 639–649. DOI: 10.1177/153537020322800601

15. Burke, V., Gracey, M. (1980) 'Effects of salicylate on intestinal absorption: in vitro and in vivo studies with enterotoxigenic micro-organisms'. *Gut* 21(8), pp. 683–688. DOI: 10.1136/gut.21.8.683

16. Schumann, K. (2001) 'Safety aspects of iron in food'. *Ann. Nutr. Metab* 45(3), pp. 91–101. DOI: 10.1159/000046713.

17. Chen, W-W., Zhang, X., Huang, W-J. (2016) 'Role of neuroinflammation in neurodegenerative diseases (Review)'. *Molecular Medicine Reports* 13(4), pp. 3391–3396. DOI: 10.3892/mmr.2016.4948

18. Albrecht, D.S., Granziera, C., Hooker, J.M., Loggia, M.L. (2016) 'In vivo imaging of human neuroinflammation', *ACS Chemical Neuroscience*, 7(4), pp. 470–483. DOI: 10.1021/acschemneuro.6b00056

19. Morris, G., Maes, M. (2013) 'A neuroimmune model of myalgic encephalomyelitis/chronic fatigue syndrome'. *Metabolic Brain Disease* 28(4), pp. 523–540. DOI: 10.1007/s11011-012-9324-8

20. Sin, D.D. (2023) 'Is long COVID an autoimmune disease?' *European Respiratory Journal* 61(1), p. 2202272.
DOI: 10.1183/13993003.02272-2022

21. Frere, J.J., *et al.* (2022) 'SARS-CoV-2 infection in hamsters and humans results in lasting and unique systemic perturbations post recovery'. *Sci. Transl. Med* 14(664), p. eabq3059. DOI: 10.1126/scitranslmed.abq3059

22. Morris, G., Berk, M., Walder, K., Maes, M. (20150 'Central pathways causing fatigue in neuro-inflammatory and autoimmune illnesses'. *BMC Medicine* 13, p. 28. DOI: 10.1186/s12916-014-0259-2

23. Gárate, I., *et al.* (2013) 'Stress-induced neuroinflammation: role of the toll-like receptor-4 pathway'. *Biological Psychiatry* 73(1), pp. 32–43.
DOI: 10.1016/j.biopsych.2012.07.005

24. Liu, J.J., Buisman-Pijlman, F., Hutchinson, M.R. (2014) 'Toll-like receptor 4: innate immune regulator of neuroimmune and neuroendocrine interactions in stress and major depressive disorder'. *Frontiers in Neuroscience* 8, p. 309.
DOI: 10.3389/fnins.2014.00309

25. Liu, Q., *et al.* (2020) 'Pathological changes in the lungs and lymphatic organs of 12 COVID-19 autopsy cases'. *National Science Review* 7(12), pp. 1868-1878.
DOI: 10.1093/nsr/nwaa247

26. Diaz, J.H. (2020) 'Hypothesis: angiotensin-converting enzyme inhibitors and

angiotensin receptor blockers may increase the risk of severe COVID-19'. *Journal of Travel Medicine* 27(3):taaa041.
DOI: 10.1093/jtm/taaa041

27. Simpson, J.B. (1981) 'The circumventricular organs and the central actions of angiotensin'. *Neuroendocrinology* 32(4), pp. 248–256.
DOI: 10.1159/000123167

28. Leitzke, M. (2023) 'Is the post-COVID-19 syndrome a severe impairment of acetylcholine-orchestrated neuromodulation that responds to nicotine administration?' *Bioelectron* 9(1), p. 2.
DOI: 10.1186/s42234-023-00104-7

29. Jett, D.A., Kuhlmann, A.C., Farmer, S.J., Guilarte, T.R. (1997) 'Age-dependent effects of developmental lead exposure on performance in the Morris water maze'. *Pharmacol. Biochem. Behav* 57(1–2), pp. 271–279.
DOI: 10.1016/s0091-3057(96)00350-4

30. Offit, K., Groeger, E., Turner, S., Wadsworth, E.A., Weiser, M.A. (2004) 'The 'duty to warn' a patient's family members about hereditary disease risks'. *JAMA* 292(12), pp. 1469–1473. DOI: 10.1001/jama.292.12.1469

31. Tilson, H.A., Mitchell, C.L. (1992) *Neurotoxicology*. New York: Raven Press.

32. Kammuller, M.E., Bloksma, N., Seinen, W. (eds) (1989) *Autoimmunity and Toxicology: Immune Disregulation Induced by Drugs and Chemicals*. Amsterdam: Elsevier.

33. Czaja, A.J., Donaldson, P.T. (2000) 'Genetic susceptibilities for immune expression and liver cell injury in autoimmune hepatitis', *Immunol. Rev.* 174, pp. 250–259. DOI: 10.1034/j.1600-0528.2002.017401.x

34. Motulsky, A.G. (1992) 'Ecogenetics: genetic predisposition to the toxic effects of chemicals'. *Am. J. Hum. Genet* 50(4), pp. 881–882.

35. Taylor, K., Pearson, M., Das, S. et al. (2023) 'Genetic risk factors for severe and fatigue dominant long COVID and commonalities with ME/CFS identified by combinatorial analysis'. *J. Transl. Med* 21(1), p. 775. DOI: 10.1186/s12967-023-04588-4

Chapter 4   Treating long COVID using the Perrin Technique™

1. Kinmonth, J.B., Sharpey-Schafer, E.P. (1959) 'Manometry of human thoracic duct'. *J. Physiol. (Lond.)* 145, p. 3.

2. Kinmonth, J.B. (1960) 'Some aspects of cardiovascular surgery'. *J. Royal*

College of Surgery Edinb. 5, pp. 287–297.

3. Browse, N.L. (1968) 'Response of lymphatics of canine hind limb to sympathetic nerve stimulation'. *J. Physiol.* 197(1), pp. 25–36. DOI: 10.1113/jphysiol.1968.sp008542

4. Kinmonth, J.B. (1982) *The Lymphatics*. 2nd edn. London: Edward Arnold, p. 80.

5. Russell, N., Low, R.N., Low, R.J., Akrami, A. (2023) 'A review of cytokine-based pathophysiology of Long COVID symptoms'. *N Front Med* 10: p. 1011936. DOI: 10.3389/fmed.2023.1011936).

6. Cruikshank, W.C. (1786) *The anatomy of Absorbing Vessels of the Human Body*. London: G. Nicoli.

7. Mascagni, P. (1787) *Vasorum Lymphaticorum Corporis Humani*. Siena, Italy: Pazzini Carli, Tabula XXVll.

8. Iliff, J. *et al.* (2012) 'A paravascular pathway facilitates CSF flow through the brain parenchyma and the clearance of interstitial solutes, including amyloid beta'. *Sci. Transl. Med.* 4(147). DOI: 10.1126/scitranslmed.3003748

9. Burnstock, G. (2007) Physiology and pathophysiology of purinergic neurotransmission. *Review Physiol Rev* 87(2): 659-797. DOI: 10.1152/physrev.00043.2006

10. Xie, L. *et al.* (2013) 'Sleep drives metabolite clearance from the adult brain'. *Science* 342(6156): pp. 373–377. DOI: 10.1126/science.1241224

11. Jason, L.A., Zinn, M.L., Zinn, M.A. (2015) 'Myalgic encephalomyelitis: symptoms and biomarkers'. Curr Neuropharmacol 13(5), pp. 701–734. DOI: 10.2174/1570159x13666150928105725

12. Lee, H., Xie, L., Yu, M., Kang, H., *et al.* (2015) 'The effect of body posture on brain glymphatic transport'. *J Neurosci* 35(31): 11034–11044.

13. Low, R.N., Low, R.J., Akrami, A. (2023) 'A review of cytokine-based pathophysiology of Long COVID symptoms'. *Front Med (Lausanne)* 10, p. 1011936. DOI: 10.3389/fmed.2023.1011936

14. Ceglarek, L., Boyman, O. (2024) 'Immune dysregulation in long COVID'. *Nat. Immunol.* 25(4), pp. 587–589. DOI: 10.1038/s41590-024-01795-z

15. Peters, V.A, Joesting, J.J., Freund, G.G. (2012) 'IL-1 receptor 2 (IL-1R2) and its role in immune regulation'. *Brain Behav. Immun.* 32, pp. 1–8. DOI: 10.1016/j.bbi.2012.11.006

16. Hives, L., Bradley, A., Richards, J., Sutton, C., *et al.* (2017) 'Can physical assessment techniques aid diagnosis in people with chronic fatigue syndrome/ myalgic encephalomyelitis? A diagnostic accuracy study'. *BMJ Open* 7(11): e017521.
    DOI: 10.1136/ bmjopen-2017-017521

17. Heald, A.H., Perrin, R., Walther, A., *et al.* (2022) 'Reducing fatigue-related symptoms in long COVID-19: a preliminary report of a lymphatic drainage intervention'. *Cardiovasc Endocrinol Metab* 11(2): e0261.
    DOI: 10.1097/XCE.0000000000000261

18. Liu, D.L., Duricka, D.L. (2022) 'Stellate ganglion block reduces symptoms of Long COVID: A case series'. *J. Neuroimmunol.* 362, p. 577784.
    DOI: 10.1016/j.jneuroim.2021.577784

19. Still, A.T. (1902) *The Philosophy and Mechanical Principles of Osteopathy.* Kansas City, Mo: Hudson-Kimberly Pub Co. Available at: http://www.interlinea. org/atstill/eBookPMPO_V2.0.pdf (Accessed: 4 May 2024).

20. Dreha-Kulaczewski, S., *et al.* (2015) 'Inspiration is the major regulator of human CSF Flow'. *Journal of Neuroscience* 35(6) pp. 2485–2491.
    DOI: 10.1523/JNEUROSCI.3246-14.2015

21. Ali, M. (2011) *The Neck Connection.* Sugar & Spice Resources Ltd.

22. Sutherland, W.G. (1939) *The Cranial Bowl.* Mankato, Minnesota: Free Press Company.

23. Sutherland, W.G. (1990) *Teachings in the Science of Osteopathy.* Edited by A.W. Wales. Fort Worth, TX: Sutherland Cranial Teaching Foundation.

24. Pessa, J.E. (2022) 'Ventricular infusion and nanoprobes identify cerebrospinal fluid and glymphatic circulation in human nerves'. *Plasr Reconstr Surg Glob Open* 10(2): e4126.

25. Pelz, H., Müller, G., Keller, M., *et al.* (2023) 'Validation of subjective manual palpation using objective physiological recordings of the cranial rhythmic impulse during osteopathic manipulative intervention'. *Sci. Rep..* 13(1), p. 6611.
    DOI: 10.1038/s41598-023-33644-8

26. Stępnik, J., Kedra, A., Czaprowski, D. (2023) 'Effects of the fourth ventricle compression technique and rib raising osteopathic technique on autonomic nervous system activity measured by heart rate variability in 35 healthy individuals'. *Med Sci Monit* 29, p. e941167-1–e941167.
    DOI: 10.12659/MSM.941167

27. Perrin, R.N., Edwards, J., Hartley, P. (1998) 'An evaluation of the effectiveness of osteopathic treatment on symptoms associated with Myalgic Encephalomyelitis: A preliminary report'. *Journal of Medical Engineering and Technology* 22(1), pp. 1-13. DOI: 10.3109/03091909809009993

28. Perrin, R.N. (2007) *The Perrin Technique: How to beat Chronic Fatigue Syndrome*. London, UK: Hammersmith Press.

29. Perrin, R.N. (2021) *The Perrin Technique: How to Diagnose and Treat Chronic Fatigue Syndrome/ME and Fibromyalgia via the Lymphatic Drainage of the Brain*. 2nd edn. London, UK: Hammersmith Health Books.

30. Perrin, R.N. (2021) *The Concise Perrin Technique: A Handbook for Patients*. London, UK: Hammersmith Health Books.

Chapter 5 The recovery process

1. Sawatsky, J. (2017) *Dancing With Elephants*. Winnipeg: Red Canoe Press, p. 204.

2. Porter, N. and Jason, L.A. (2022) 'Mindfulness meditation interventions for long Covid: biobehavioral gene expression and neuroimmune functioning'. *Neuropsychiatr Dis Treat* 18, pp. 2599–2626. DOI: 10.2147/NDT.S379653

3. Perrin, R.N., Edwards, J., Hartley, P. (1998) 'An evaluation of the effectiveness of osteopathic treatment on symptoms associated with Myalgic Encephalomyelitis. A preliminary report'. *Journal of Medical Engineering and Technology* 22(1), pp. 1– 3. DOI: 10.3109/03091909809009993

4. Lundberg, G. (2024) 'Long COVID: another great pretender', *Medscape*, 9 Feb. Available at: https://www.medscape.com/viewarticle/1000083?form=fpf (Accessed: 26 March 2024).

Chapter 6 Can long COVID be cured?

1. Møllgård, K., Beinlich, F., Kusk, P., *et al.* (2023) 'A mesothelium divides the subarachnoid space into functional compartments'. *Science* 379(6627), pp. 84-88. DOI: 10.1126/science.adc8810

2. Grach, S.L., Ganesh, R., Messina, S.A., *et al.* (2022) 'Post-COVID-19 syndrome: persistent neuroimaging changes and symptoms 9 months after initial infection'. *BMJ Case Rep* 15(4), p. e248448. DOI:10.1136/bcr-2021-248448

3. Iliff, J., *et al*l. (2012) 'A paravascular pathway facilitates CSF flow through the brain parenchyma and the clearance of interstitial solutes, including amyloid beta'. *Sci. Transl. Med.*, 4(147), p. 147ra111. DOI: 10.1126/scitranslmed.3003748

4. Thapilaya, K., *et al.* (2023) 'Brainstem volume changes in myalgic encephalomyelitis/chronic fatigue syndrome and long COVID patients'. *Frontiers in Neuroscience* 17, p. 1125208. DOI: 10.3389/fnins.2023.1125208

5. Mestre, H., Tithof, J., Du, T., *et al.* (2018) 'Flow of cerebrospinal fluid is driven by arterial pulsations and is reduced in hypertension'. *Nat. Commun* 9(1), p. 4878. DOI: 10.1038/s41467-018-07318-3

6. Pessa, J.E. (2023) 'Identification of a novel path for cerebrospinal fluid (CSF) drainage of the human brain'. *PLoS ONE* 18(5), p. e0285269. DOI: 10.1371/journal.pone.0285269

7. Pessa, J. E. (2022) 'Ventricular infusion and nanoprobes identify cerebrospinal fluid and glymphatic circulation in human nerves'. *Plasr. Reconstr. Surg. Glob. Open* 10(2), p. e4126. DOI: 10.1097/GOX.0000000000004126

8. Oaklander, A.L., *et al.* (2022) 'Peripheral neuropathy evaluations of patients with prolonged long COVID'. *Neurol Neuroimmunol Neuroinflamm* 9(3), p. e1146. DOI: 10.1212/NXI.0000000000001146

9. Yoon, J.H., *et al.* (2024) 'Nasopharyngeal lymphatic plexus is a hub for cerebrospinal fluid drainage'. *Nature* 625(7996), p. 768-777. DOI: 10.1038/s41586-023-06899-4

10. Spera, I., Proulx, S.T. (2024) 'A nasal hub for cerebrospinal fluid clearance'. *Nat. Cardiovasc. Res* 3, pp. 98-99. DOI: 10.1038/s44161-024-00423-1

11. Chen, C., *et al.* (2022) 'Adenosine downregulates the activities of glutamatergic neurons in the paraventricular hypothalamic nucleus required for sleep'. *Front. Neurosci* 16, p. 907155. DOI: 10.3389/fnins.2022.907155

12. McCormick, D.A., Bal, T. (1994) 'Sensory gating mechanisms of the thalamus', *Current Opinion in Neurobiology*, 4(4), pp. 550-556. DOI: 10.1016/0959-4388(94)90056-6

13. Walker, M. (2018) *Why We Sleep: The New Science of Sleep and Dreams*. London, UK: Penguin Books.

14. Xie, L., *et al.* (2013) 'Sleep drives metabolite clearance from the adult brain'. *Science* 342, pp. 373–377. DOI: 10.1126/science.1241224

15. Fultz, N.E., *et al.* (2019) 'Coupled electrophysiological, hemodynamic, and cerebrospinal fluid oscillations in human sleep'. *Science* 366, pp. 628–631. DOI: 10.1126/science.aax544

16. Lewis, L. (2021) 'The interconnected causes and consequences of sleep in the brain'. *Science* 374(6567), pp. 564–568. DOI: 10.1126/science.abi8375

17. Walker, M. (2018) 'Dreaming – the soothing balm' in *Why We Sleep*. London, UK: Penguin Books, pp. 205–207.

18. Destexhe, A, Foubert, L.A. (2022) 'A method to convert neural signals into sound sequences'. *J. Acoust Soc Am* 151(6), p. 3685. DOI: 10.1121/10.0011549

19. Ray, C., Weir, W.R.C., Phillips, L., Cullen, S. (1992) 'Development of a measure of symptoms in chronic fatigue syndrome: the profile of fatigue related symptoms (PFRS)'. *Psychol Health* 7, pp. 27–43. DOI:10.1080/08870449208404293

20. Perrin, R., Riste, L., Hann, M., Heald, A.H. (2024) 'Deep sleep improved by a manual therapy aimed at aiding glymphatic drainage in Long COVID: A case study'. *Fatigue: Biomedicine, Health & Behavior* (Accepted, awaiting publication)

21. Lee, H., *et al.* (2015) 'The effect of body posture on brain glymphatic transport'. *J. Neurosci* 35(31), pp.11034–11044. DOI: 10.1523/JNEUROSCI.1625-15.2015

22. Person, E., *et al.* (2015) 'A novel sleep positioning device reduces gastroesophageal reflux: a randomized controlled trial'. *J. Clin. Gastroenterol* 49(8), pp. 655–659. DOI: 10.1097/MCG.0000000000000359

23. Iliff, J., Wang, M., Liao, Y., Plogg, B., *et al.* (2012) 'Paravascular pathway facilitates CSF flow through the brain parenchyma and the clearance of

interstitial solutes, including amyloid beta'. *Sci Transl Med* 4 (147), p. 147ra111. DOI: 10.1126/scitranslmed.3003748

24. Thapaliya, K., Marshall-Gradisnik, S., Barth, M., Eaton-Fitch, N., Barnden, L. (2023) 'Brainstem volume changes in ME/CFS and Long Covid patients'. *Frontiers of Neuroscience* 17, p. 1125208.
    DOI. 10.3389/fnins.2023.1125208

25. Perrin, R.N. (2005) *The involvement of cerebrospinal fluid and lymphatic drainage in chronic fatigue syndrome/ME*, PhD Thesis, University of Salford.

26. Goldstein, J. (1993) *Chronic Fatigue Syndromes: The Limbic Hypothesis*. New York, NY, US: The Haworth Medical Press.

27. McKeown-Eyssen, G., Baines, C., Cole, D.E., Riley, *et al.* (2004) 'Case-control study of genotypes in multiple chemical sensitivity: CYP2D6, NAT1, NAT2, PON1, PON2 and MTHFR'. *Int J Epidemiol* 33(5), pp. 971-978.
    DOI: 10.1093/ije/dyh251

28. Mackey, A. (2021) 'A paradigm for post-Covid-19 fatigue syndrome analogous to ME/CFS'. *Front Neurol* 12, p. 701419.
    DOI: 10.3389/fneur.2021.701419

29. Małkowska, P., Sawczuk, M. (2023) 'Cytokines as biomarkers for evaluating physical exercise in trained and non-trained individuals: a narrative review'. *Int. J. Mol. Sci* 24(13), p. 11156.
    DOI: 10.3390/ijms241311156

30. Dworak, M., Die,l P., Voss, S., Hollmann, W., Strüder, H.K. 'Intense exercise increases adenosine concentrations in rat brain: implications for a homeostatic sleep drive'. *Neuroscience* 150(4), pp. 789–79.
    DOI: 10.1016/j.neuroscience.2007.09.062

31. Allado, E., *et al.* (2022) 'Is there a relationship between hyperventilation syndrome and history of acute SARS-CoV-2 infection? A cross-sectional study'. *Healthcare (Basel)* 10(11), p. 2154.
    DOI: 10.3390/healthcare10112154

32. Bohr, C. (1904) 'Theoretische Behandlung der quantitativen Verhättnisse der Kohlensäurebindiung des Hämoglobins'. *Centralblatt für Physiol* 24, p. 24.

33. Harman, D. (1956) 'Aging: a theory based on free radical and radiation chemistry'. *Gerontol* 11(3), pp. 298–300. DOI: 10.1093/geronj/11.3.298

34. Kodama, M., Kodama, T., Murakami, M. (1996) 'The value of the dehydroepiandrosterone-annexed vitamin C infusion treatment in the clinical

control of chronic fatigue syndrome (CFS). II. Characterization of CFS patients with special reference to their response to a new vitamin C infusion treatment'. *In Vivo*, 10(6), pp. 585–596.

35. Thomas, L.D., Elinder, C.G., Tiselius, H.G., Wolk, A., Akesson, A. (2013) 'Ascorbic acid supplements and kidney stone incidence among men: a prospective study'. *JAMA Intern Med* 173(5), pp. 386–388. DOI: 10.1001/jamainternmed.2013.2296

36. Jiang, K., Tang, K., Liu, H., Xu, H., Ye, Z., Chen, Z. (2019) 'Ascorbic acid supplements and kidney stones incidence among men and women: a systematic review and meta-analysis'. *Urol. J* 216(2), pp. 115–120. DOI: 10.22037/uj.v0i0.4275

37. Pall, M.L. (2000) 'Elevated, sustained peroxynitrite levels as the cause of chronic fatigue syndrome'. *Med. Hypotheses* 54(1), pp. 115–125. DOI: 10.1054/mehy.1998.0825

38. Pall, M.L., Satterlee, J.D. (2001) 'Elevated nitric oxide/peroxynitrite mechanism for the common etiology of multiple chemical sensitivity, chronic fatigue syndrome and posttraumatic stress disorder'. *Ann NY Acad Sci* 933, pp. 323–329. DOI: 10.1111/j.1749-6632.2001.tb05836.x

39. Stringer, E.A., *et al.* (2013) 'Daily cytokine fluctuations, driven by leptin, are associated with fatigue severity in chronic fatigue syndrome: evidence of inflammatory pathology'. *J. Transl. Med* 11, p. 93. DOI: 10.1186/1479-5876-11-93

40. Montaya, J.G., Holmes, T.H., *et al.* (2017) 'Cytokine signature associated with disease severity in chronic fatigue syndrome patients'. *Proc Natl Acad Sci* 114(34), p. E7150–E7158. DOI: 10.1073/pnas.1710519114

41. Lazarus, M., *et al.* (2007) 'EP3 prostaglandin receptors in the median preoptic nucleus are critical for fever responses'. *Nat. Neurosci* 10(9), pp. 1131–1133. DOI: 10.1038/nn1949

42. Al-Hakeim, H.K., Al-Rubaye, H.T., Al-Hadrawi, D.S., *et al.* (2023) 'Long-COVID post-viral chronic fatigue and affective symptoms are associated with oxidative damage, lowered antioxidant defenses and inflammation: a proof of concept and mechanism study'. *Mol. Psychiatry* 28, pp. 564–578. DOI: 10.1038/s41380-022-01836-9

43. Gil, A., Hoag, G.E., Salerno, J.P., Hornig, M., Klimas, N., Selin, L.K. (2024)

'Identification of CD8 T-cell dysfunction associated with symptoms in myalgic encephalomyelitis/chronic fatigue syndrome (ME/CFS) and Long COVID and treatment with a nebulized antioxidant/anti-pathogen agent in a retrospective case series'. *Brain, Behavior, & Immunity Health* 36, p. 100720. DOI: 10.1016/j.bbih.2023.100720

44. Medinger, G., Altman, D. (2022) The Long Covid Handbook, London, UK: Penguin Random House, p. 7.

45. Riste, L., Perrin, R.N., Heald, A.H. *et al.* (in press) 'Testing the feasibility of the Perrin Technique self-help intervention to reduce fatigue-related symptoms among patients with long COVID-19 in general practice: Experiences from our randomised controlled trial (RCT)'

Chapter 7   Self-help advice

1. Nestor, J. (2021) *Breath: The New Science of a Lost Art*. London, UK: Penguin Life.

2. Ramchandra, R., *et al.* (2005) 'Nitric oxide and sympathetic nerve activity in the control of blood pressure'. *Clin. Exp. Pharmacol. Physiol* 32(5-6), pp. 440-6. DOI: 10.1111/j.1440-1681.2005.04208.x

3. Eby, G.A. (2006) 'Strong humming for one hour daily to terminate chronic rhinosinusitis in four days: A case report and hypothesis for action by stimulation of endogenous nasal nitric oxide production'. *Medical Hypotheses* 66(4), pp. 851-854. DOI: 10.1016/j.mehy.2005.11.035

Chapter 8   Other treatments that may help

1. Gross, M., *et al.* (2023) 'What do I need to know about long-Covid-related fatigue, brain fog, and mental health changes?' *Arch Phys Med Rehabil* 104(6), pp. 996–1002. DOI: 10.1016/j.apmr.2022.11.021

2. Agombar, F. (2022) *Beat Fatigue with Yoga*. 2nd revised edn. London, UK: Cherry Red Books.

3. Lee, H. *et al.* (2015) *'The effect of body posture on brain glymphatic transport'*. *J Neurosci* 35(31), pp. 11034–11044.

DOI: 10.1523/JNEUROSCI.1625-15.2015

4. Person, E., *et al.* (2015) 'A novel sleep positioning device reduces gastroesophageal reflux: a randomized controlled trial'. *J Clin Gastroenterol* 49(8), pp. 655–659.
   DOI: 10.1097/MCG.0000000000000359

5. Crinnion, W. (2011) 'Sauna as a valuable clinical tool for cardiovascular, autoimmune, toxicant-induced and other chronic health problems'. *Alternative Medicine Review* 16(3), pp. 215–225.

6. Walther, A., Grub, J., Tsar, S., Ehlert, U., Heald, A., Perrin, R., *et al.* (2023) 'Status loss due to COVID-19, traditional masculinity, and their association with recent suicide attempts and suicidal ideation'. *Psychology of Men & Masculinities* 24(1), pp. 47–62.
   DOI: 10.1037/men0000408

7. Woodward, S.F., *et al.* (2022) 'Anxiety, Post-COVID-19 syndrome-related depression, and suicidal thoughts and behaviors in Covid-19 survivors: cross-sectional study'. *JMIR Form Res* 6(10), p. e36656.
   DOI: 10.2196/36656

8. Efstathiou, V., *et al.* (2022) 'Long COVID and neuropsychiatric manifestations (Review)'. *Exp Ther Med* 23(5), p. 363.
   DOI: 10.3892/etm.2022.11290

9. Sher, L. (2023) 'Long COVID and the risk of suicide'. *Gen Hosp Psychiatry* 80, pp. 66–67. DOI: 10.1016/j.genhosppsych.2022.12.001

10. Lynch, S., Seth, R., Montgomery, S. (1991) 'Antidepressant therapy in the chronic fatigue syndrome'. *British Journal of General Practice* 41(349), pp. 339–342.

11. Wong, A.C., *et al.* (2023) 'Serotonin reduction in post-acute sequelae of viral infection'. *Cell* 186(22), pp. 4851–4867.
    DOI: 10.1016/j.cell.2023.09.013

12. Barandouzi, Z.A., Lee, J., del Carmen Rosas, M., *et al.* (2022) 'Associations of neurotransmitters and the gut microbiome with emotional distress in mixed type of irritable bowel syndrome'. *Sci Rep* 12(1), p. 1648.
    DOI: 10.1038/s41598-022-05756-0

13. The Happiness Trap Newsletter (n.d.) *Interview with Steven Hayes*. Available at: https://thehappinesstrap.com/upimages/Steve_Hayes_Interview.pdf (Accessed: 6 May 2024).

14. Hughes, L.S., *et al.* (2017) 'Acceptance and commitment therapy (ACT) for chronic pain: a systematic review and meta-analyses'. *Clin J Pain* 33(6), pp. 552–568. DOI: 10.1097/AJP.0000000000000425

15. Hayes, S.C., Strosahl, K., Wilson, K.G. (1999) *Acceptance and commitment therapy: An experiential approach to behavior change.* Hove, US: Guilford Press.

16. Hayes, S.C., Smith, S. (2005) *Get out of your mind and your life – The new acceptance and commitment therapy.* Oakland, CA, US: New Harbinger.

17. Association for Contextual and Behavioral Science (ACBS) (2021) *State of the ACT evidence.* Available at: https://contextualscience.org/state_of_the_act_evidence (Accessed: 6 May 2024).

18. Elvis, A.M., Ekta, J.S. (2011) 'Ozone therapy: a clinical review'. *J Nat Sci Biol Med* 2(1), pp. 66–70. DOI: 10.4103/0976-9668.82319

19. Hsu, H.H., Leung, W.H., Hu, G.C. (2016) 'Treatment of irritable bowel syndrome with a novel colonic irrigation system: a pilot study'. *Tech Coloproctol* 20(8), pp. 551-557. DOI: 10.1007/s10151-016-1491-x

20. Stavrakis, S., Elkholey, K., Morris, L., Niewiadomska, M., Asad, Z.U.A., Humphrey, M.B. (2022) 'Neuromodulation of inflammation to treat heart failure with preserved ejection fraction: a pilot randomized clinical trial', *Journal of the American Heart Association.* 11(3), p. e023582.
DOI: 10.1161/JAHA.121.023582

21. Seitz, T., Szeles, J.C., Kitzberger, R., Holbik, J., *et al*, E..(2022) 'Percutaneous auricular vagus nerve stimulation reduces inflammation in critical Covid-19 patients'. *Front Physiol*13, p. 897257.
DOI: 10.3389/fphys.2022.897257

22. Tornero, C., *et al.* (2022) 'Non-invasive vagus nerve stimulation for COVID-19: results from a randomized controlled trial'. *Front Neurol* 13, p. 820864.
DOI: 10.3389/fneur.2022.820864

23. Thakkar, V.J., Richardson, Z.A., Dang, A., Centanni, T. (2021) 'Improvement of memory-based reading recall using transcutaneous auricular vagus nerve stimulation'. *Behavioural Brain Research* 438, p. 114164.
DOI: 10.1016/j.bbr.2022.114164

24. Thakkar, V.J., Engelhart, A.S., Khodaparast, N., Abadzi, H. Centanni, T.M. (2020) 'Transcutaneous auricular vagus nerve stimulation enhances learning of novel letter–sound relationships in adults'. *Brain Stimulation* 13(6), pp. 1813–

1820. DOI: 10.1016/j.brs.2020.10.012

25. Nguyen, T.C., Kiss, J.E., Goldman, J.R., Carcillo, J.A. (2012) 'The role of plasmapheresis in critical illness'. *Crit. Care Clin* 28(3), pp. 453–468. DOI: 10.1016/j.ccc.2012.04.009

26. Scheibenbogen, C., *et al. (2018) 'Immunoadsorption to remove ß2 adrenergic receptor antibodies in Chronic Fatigue Syndrome ME/CFS'. PLoS One* 13(3), p. e0193672. DOI: 10.1371/journal.pone.0193672

27. Younger, J., Mackey, S. (2009) 'Fibromyalgia symptoms are reduced by low-dose naltrexone: a pilot study'. *Pain Med* 10(4), pp. 663–672. DOI: 10.1111/j.1526-4637.2009.00613.x

28. Metyas, S., Chen, C.L., Yeter, K., Solyman, J., Arkfeld, D.G. (2018) 'Low dose naltrexone in the treatment of fibromyalgia'. *Curr. Rheumatol. Rev* 14(2), pp. 177–180. DOI: 10.2174/1573397113666170321120329

29. Eisenstein T.K. (2019) 'The role of opioid receptors in immune system function front'. *Immunol* 10, p. 2904. DOI:10.3389/fimmu.2019.02904

30. Younger, J., Parkitny, L., Mclain, D. (2014) 'The use of low-dose naltrexone (LDN) as a novel anti-inflammatory treatment for chronic pain'. *Clin Rheumatol* 33(4), pp. 451–459. DOI: 10.1007/s10067-014-2517-2

31. Putrino D. (2023) *Long COVID and its neighbors: understanding the pathobiology of long COVID and other post acute infection syndromes (PAIS).* Plenary presentation at the International Association CFS/ME (IACFS/ME) Conference, Stony Brook University, NY, July 2023.

32. 32. Heald, A.H., Perrin, R., Walther, A., *et al.* (2022) 'Reducing fatigue-related symptoms in long COVID-19: a preliminary report of a lymphatic drainage intervention'. *Cardiovasc Endocrinol Metab* 11(2), p. e0261. DOI: 10.1097/XCE.0000000000000261

33. Halpin, S., O'Connor, R., Sivan, M. (2021) 'Long COVID and chronic COVID syndromes'. *J Med Virol* 93, pp.1242–1243. DOI: 10.1002/jmv.26587

Chapter 9 Diet and supplements

1. Myhill, S., Robinson, C. (2022) *Paleo-Ketogenic: The Why and The How.* London, UK: Hammersmith Health Books.

2. Kassam, S., Kassam, Z. (2022) *Eating Plant-Based*. London, UK: Hammersmith Health Books.

3. Chang, K., *et al.* (2023) 'Ultra-processed food consumption, cancer risk and cancer mortality: a large-scale prospective analysis within the UK Biobank'. *EClinical Medicine* 56, p. 101840. DOI: 10.1016/j.eclinm.2023.10184

4. Lea, G. (2021) 'Could a glass of wine diagnose long COVID?' *KevinMD.com* 12 March. Available at: https://www.kevinmd.com/post-author/georgia-lea (Accessed: 7 May 2024).

5. Farah, Y., *et al.* (2023) 'Adverse events following COVID-19 mRNA vaccines: A systematic review of cardiovascular complication, thrombosis, and thrombocytopenia'. *Immun Inflamm Dis* 11(3), p. e807. DOI: 10.1002/iid3.807

6. Dyer, C. (2023) 'Patients launch legal action against AstraZeneca over its covid-19 vaccine'. *BMJ* 380, p. 725. DOI: 10.1136/bmj.p725

7. Barletta, A., *et al.* (2022) 'Coenzyme Q10+alpha lipoic acid for chronic COVID syndrome'. *Clin Exp Med* 23(3), pp. 667–678. DOI: 10.1007/s10238-022-00871-8

8. Werbach, M. (1998) 'Nutritional strategies for treating chronic fatigue syndrome'. *Alternative Medicine Review* 5(2), pp. 93–108.

9. Cox, I.M., Campbell, M.J., Dowson, D. (1991) 'Red blood cell magnesium and chronic fatigue syndrome'. *Lancet* 337(8744), pp. 757–760. DOI: 10.1016/0140-6736(91)91371-z

10. Russell, I.J., *et al.* (1995) 'Treatment of fibromyalgia syndrome with Super Malic: a randomized, double blind, placebo controlled, crossover pilot study'. *J Rheumatol* 22(5), pp. 953–958.

11. Fulgenzi, A., Vietti, D., Ferrero, M.E. (2014) 'Aluminium involvement in neurotoxicity'. *BioMed Research International* 2014, p. 758323. DOI:10.1155/2014/758323

12. Marten, B., Pfeuffer, M., Schrezenmeir, J. (2006) 'Medium-chain triglycerides'. *International Dairy Journal* 16(11), pp. 1374 - 1382.

13. Tan, Z., *et al.* (2011) 'Removal of elemental mercury by bamboo charcoal impregnated with H 2O 2'. *Fuel* 90(4), pp. 1471–1475.

14. Regland, B., Forsmark, S., Halaouate, L., *et al.* (2015) 'Response to vitamin B12 and folic acid in myalgic encephalomyelitis and fibromyalgia'. *PloS One* 10(4), p. e0124648.

DOI: 10.1371/journal.pone.0124648

15. Tsivgoulis, G., Fragkou, P.C., Karofylakis, E., *et al.* (2021) 'Hypothyroidism is associated with prolonged COVID-19-induced anosmia: a case–control study'. *Journal of Neurology, Neurosurgery & Psychiatry* 92, pp. 911–912. DOI: 10.1136/jnnp-2021-326587

16. Vanderpump, M.P., Lazarus, J.A., *et al.* (2011) 'Iodine status of UK schoolgirls: a cross-sectional survey'. *Lancet* 377(9782), pp. 2007–2012. DOI: 10.1016/S0140-6736(11)60693-4

17. Rowe, P., *et al.* (1995) 'Is neurally-mediated hypotension an unrecognised cause of chronic fatigue?' *Lancet* 345(8950), pp. 623–624. DOI: 10.1016/s0140-6736(95)90525-1

18. Castro-Marrero, J., *et al.* (2018) 'Low omega-3 index and polyunsaturated fatty acid status in patients with chronic fatigue syndrome/myalgic encephalomyelitis'. *Prostaglandins, Leukotrienes and Essential Fatty Acids* 139, pp. 20–24. DOI: 10.1016/j.plefa.2018.11.006

19. Puri, B.K., Counsell, S.J., Zaman, R., Main, J., *et al.* (20020 'Relative increase in choline in the occipital cortex in chronic fatigue syndrome'. *Acta Psychiatr Scand* 106(3), pp. 224–226. DOI: 10.1034/j.1600-0447.2002.01300.x

20. Kopańska, M., *et al.* (2022) 'Disorders of the cholinergic system in COVID-19 era—a review of the latest research'. *Int J Mol Sci* 23(2), p. 672. DOI: 10.3390/ijms23020672

21. Ren, H., *et al.* (2017) 'Omega-3 polyunsaturated fatty acids promote amyloid-β clearance from the brain through mediating the function of the glymphatic system'. *FASEB* 31(1), pp. 282–293. DOI: 10.1096/fj.201600896

22. Keshavarz, M., Showraki, A., Emamghoreishi, M. (2013) 'Anticonvulscent effect of guifenesin against pentylenetetrazol-induced seizure in mice'. *Iran J Med Sci* 38(2), pp. 116–121.

23. Karosanidze, I., *et al.* (2022) 'Efficacy of adaptogens in patients with long COVID-19: A randomized, quadruple-blind, placebo-controlled trial'. *Pharmaceuticals (Basel)* 15(3), p. 345. DOI: 10.3390/ph15030345

24. Rathi, A., Jadhav, S.B., Shah, N. (2021) 'A randomized controlled trial of the efficacy of systemic enzymes and probiotics in the resolution of post-COVID

fatigue'. *Medicines (Basel)* 8(9), p. 47.
DOI: 10.3390/medicines8090047

25. Glynne, P., Tahmasebi, N., Gant, V., *et al.* (2022) 'Long COVID following mild SARS-CoV-2 infection: characteristic T cell alterations and response to antihistamines'. *Journal of Investigative Medicine* 70(1), pp. 61-67.
DOI: 10.1136/jim-2021-002051

26. Bent, S., *et al.* (2006) 'Valerian for sleep: a systematic review and meta-analysis'. *Am J Med* 119(12), p. 1005–1012.
DOI: 10.1016/j.amjmed.2006.02.026

27. Wintergerst, E.S., Maggini, S., Hornig, D.H.(2006) 'Immune-enhancing role of vitamin C and zinc and effect on clinical conditions'. *Ann Nutr Metab* 50(2), pp.85-94. DOI: 10.1159/000090495

28. Okhuarobo, A., *et al.* (2014) 'Harnessing the medicinal properties of Andrographis paniculata for diseases and beyond: a review of its phytochemistry and pharmacology'. *Asian Pac J Trop Dis* 4(3), pp. 213–222.
DOI: 10.1016/S2222-1808(14)60509-0

29. Yanuck, S.F., *et al.* (2020) 'Evidence supporting a phased immuno-physiological approach to COVID-19 from prevention through recovery'. *Integr Med (Encinitas)* 19(Suppl 1), pp. 8–35.

30. David, A.V.A., Arulmoli, R., Parasuraman, S. (2016) 'Overviews of biological importance of Quercetin: a bioactive flavonoid'. *Pharmacogn Rev* 10(20), pp. 84–89. DOI: 10.4103/0973-7847

31. Bouic, P.J., Lamprecht, J.H. (1999) 'Plant sterols and sterolins: a review of their immune-modulating properties'. *Altern Med Rev* 4(3), pp. 170-7.

32. Ankri, S., Mirelman, D. (1999) 'Antimicrobial properties of allicin from garlic'. *Microbes Infect* 1(2), pp. 125–129.
DOI: 10.1016/s1286-4579(99)80003-3

33. Ionescu, G., *et al.* (1989) 'Oral citrus seed extract in atopic eczema: in vitro and in vivo studies on intestinal microflora'. *Journal of Orthomolecular Medicine* 5(3), pp. 155–157.

34. Lucretius (1963) *De Rerum Natura*. 2nd edn. Cyril Bailey (ed.). Oxford: Oxford Classical Texts.

Appendix   Frequently asked questions

1. Fahdah, A., *et al.* (2019) 'The effect of smartphone usage at bedtime on sleep quality among Saudi non-medical staff at King Saud University Medical City'. *J. Family Med. Prim. Care* 8(6), pp.1953–1957.
    DOI: 10.4103/jfmpc.jfmpc_269_19

2. Machado, K., Ayuk, P. (2023) 'Post-COVID-19 condition and pregnancy'. *Case Rep. Women's Health* 37, p. e00458.
    DOI: 10.1016/j.crwh.2022.e00458

3. Schacterle, R.S., Komaroff, A.L. (2004) 'A Comparison of Pregnancies That Occur Before and After the Onset of Chronic Fatigue Syndrome'. *Arch Intern Med* 164(4): pp. 401–404.

4. Allen, V. (2024) 'Burning scented candles could be harmful for your health and increase the risk of migraines or respiratory diseases, expert warns', *Daily Mail Online*, 1 Jan. Available at:
    www.dailymail.co.uk/news/article-12917289 (Accessed: 13 May 2024).

5. Iliff, J., *et al.* (2012) 'A paravascular pathway facilitates CSF flow through the brain parenchyma and the clearance of interstitial solutes, including amyloid beta', *Sci. Transl. Med.*, 4(147), p. 147ra111.
    DOI: 10.1126/scitranslmed.3003748

6. Gibbs, D. (2024) *Dispatches from the Land of Alzheimer's*. Cambridge: Cambridge University Press.

7. Xie, L., Kang, H., Xu, Q., Chen, M.J., *et al.* (2013) 'Sleep drives metabolite clearance from the adult brain'. *Science* 342(6156), pp. 373–377.
    DOI: 10.1126/science.1241224

8. Lourens, G.B., Ferrell, D.K. (2019) 'Lymphatic filariasis'. *Nursing Clin North Am* 54(2), pp. 181-192. DOI: 10.1016/j.cnur.2019.02.007

9. Trincot, C.E., Caron, K.M. (2019) 'Lymphatic function and dysfunction in the context of sex differences'. *ACS Pharmacology & Translational Science* 2(5), pp. 311-324. DOI: 10.1021/acsptsci.9b00051

10. Lim, C., Leung, A.K.C., Leong, K.F., Lam, J.M. (2023) 'Primary lymphedema in a pediatric patient'. *Consultant* 63(2), p. e6.

11. Berton, M., Lorette, G., Baulieu, F., Lagrue, E., Blesson, S., Cambazard, F. and Maruani, A. (2015) 'Generalized lymphedema associated with neurologic signs (GLANS) syndrome: a new entity?' *Journal of the American Academy of*

Dermatology 72(2), 333–339.

DOI: 10.1016/j.jaad.2014.10.033

12. Keith, L. (2021) *The Lymphatic Code: Using a ketogenic lifestyle to enjoy a robust lymphatic system that promotes overall health and wellness.* Cheyenne, WY, US: Gutsy Badger Pub.

13. Heald, A.H., Perrin, R., Walther, A., *et al.* (2022) 'Reducing fatigue-related symptoms in Long COVID-19: a preliminary report of a lymphatic drainage intervention'. *Cardiovasc Endocrinol Metab* 11(2), p. e0261.

DOI: 10.1097/XCE.0000000000000261

Index

Also from Hammersmith Health Books...
... books about Pacing

Fighting Fatigue

A practical guide to managing the symptoms of CFS/ME
By Sue Pemberton, Catherine Berry and Janie Spencer

Our classic guide to pacing that has been recommended by occupational therapists
and specialist centres for chronic fatigue since 2006.

The Fatigue Book

Chronic fatigue syndrome and long COVID fatigue: Practical tips for recovery
By Lydia Rolley

'I wholeheartedly and highly recommend this book for those seeking to find a way through
the weightiness of fatigue in a gentle, strategically paced and personally meaningful way.'
Suzanne Elizabeth Davis, Physiotherapist and Family Therapist

Rest-Do Days

How to live with fatigue and get things done
. By Wendy Bryant

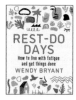

A practical guide to finding a balance between resting and doing so that readers can recharge
their energy levels and also do the things that are important to them.

Also by Dr Raymond Perrin

The Perrin Technique Second Edition

How to diagnose and treat chronic fatigue syndrome/ME and fibromyalgia via the lymphatic drainage of the brain

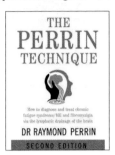

'For anyone who is involved in the diagnosis and management of ME/CFS, this is an essential read and a seminal reference text.' Dr Adrian Heald, Consultant Physician, Salford Royal Hospital, UK

The Concise Perrin Technique

A handbook for patients
A practical companion to The Perrin Technique 2nd Edition

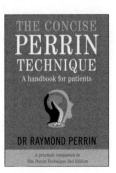

The practical guide for ME/CFS patients who want only a concise overview of the 'why' of the Perrin Technique but full details of the 'how'

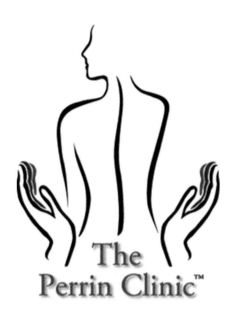

The Perrin Clinic is dedicated to helping all those with long COVID, ME/CFS, FMS and other related disorders using The Perrin Technique™

The Perrin Clinic is also committed to training and monitoring practitioners who have been licensed to treat patients with the Perrin Technique™

Only licensed practitioners may use the Perrin Technique™ name and logo as shown below:

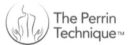

To find your nearest licensed practitioner visit:
www.theperrintechnique.com

pr@theperrinclinic.com